SWALLOWED BY A JAGUAR

A Mother's Memoir on the Loss of an Adult Child

Deborah Pearcey, Amber Landgraff
and Michelle Retterath

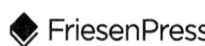 FriesenPress

One Printers Way
Altona, MB R0G 0B0
Canada

www.friesenpress.com

ISBN
978-1-03-832186-2 (Hardcover)
978-1-03-832185-5 (Paperback)
978-1-03-832187-9 (eBook)

1. BIOGRAPHY & AUTOBIOGRAPHY, PERSONAL MEMOIRS

Distributed to the trade by The Ingram Book Company

Swallowed

by a Jaguar

Deborah Pearcey

With Amber Landgraff and Michelle Retterath

"History is not what we are told but what we tell . . . We choose what we need to tell a story, hoping that it will have a beginning, middle, and end. We hope that the result will be coherence. We create reality through words. We invent arguments for our past and tell the reader or listener this is what happened."

—Alberto Manguel in the foreword of Findlay's Final Last Words, 2005

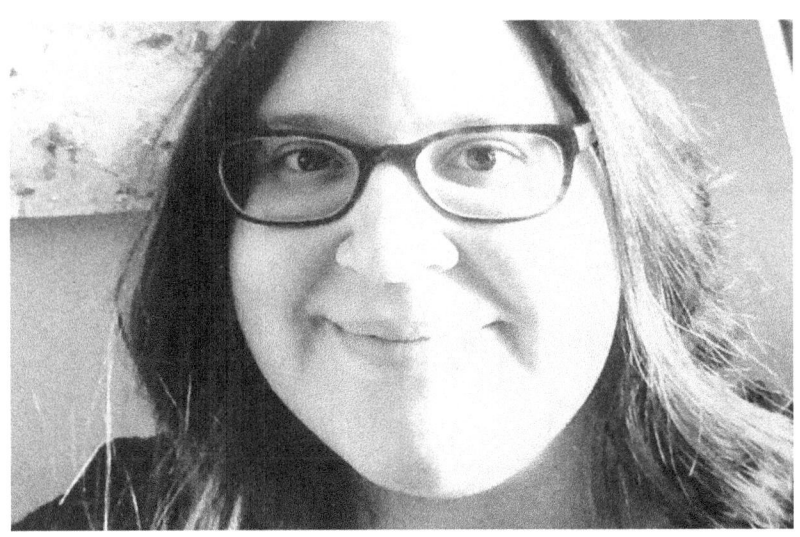

Miss. A. Landgraff
345 Rankin Dr.
Burlington, Ont.
L7N2B2

Mr, Mrs. D. Landgraff
345 Rankin Dr,
Burlington, Ont.
L7N2B2

CANADA

In 1992, an envelope arrived in the mailbox with a letter enclosed. It was supposed to be a letter by the future Amber. The Amber who was an adult. The paper was crumpled, the edges torn, and red marks slashed down the page. Then, the sheets were smoothed out as best they could be, folded, and put into the envelope. I came home from work that day not knowing that a letter would be arriving for me from my nine-year-old daughter. I cannot reproduce the paper well enough to show the actual letter, so I have retyped it.

May 29, 1992

Dear Mom:

I'm writing to you from the Amazon.
Some hunters mistook me for a jaguar and are trying to track me down.
The rainforest is beautiful, but I wouldn't like to live here.

I saw a toucan, macaw, and cook-of-the-rock.

Mom, I am sending you my love.

Today, I saw a monkey who was simply insane.

At night, I hope it's going to be peaceful, or I won't get any sleep.

I just saw a tree frog. It might be the mother. I don't know, but it was with its babies.

I don't know why people want to cut down the rainforest, but I think it is too beautiful to cut down.

Mom! I just came face to face with a jaguar. Get me out of here! I have to write the rest of this letter inside the jaguar. Don't blame me if you never get this letter. I just heard some rumbling. He just threw up.

Love,

Amber

P.S. Get me out of here and I love you.

During the hospital stay, I thought of this letter often, and I had imagined Amber to be the age she was then, thirty-four, when the letter was supposed to happen. I thought the fears for Amber's safety had become a reality of which I never could have imagined. Carcinoma was the jaguar, and Amber was being swallowed by it, and this time there was no saving her.

Imagine a young woman full of life and creative spirit. I adored Amber. She taught me so much, and she made me braver because I had to show her that she could accomplish something even though she was afraid, and I was afraid. I did those things anyway.

I truly believe that we organize thoughts in our brain by story. I find that if I can attach the information into a story, I remember it better. I think it also makes more sense and it brings me further insight. Kessler said that stories give shape to the randomness of death, a randomness which is very hard for the brain (2019). I also believe in narrative therapy. I set out with this story wanting to get the story onto paper. I hoped it would help me stop ruminating and grieving. I began to try and give meaning to Amber's death, and meaning and hope to my life. You will find that I frequently use the terms: "I didn't realize," "didn't know," or "forgot." I added an essay and quotations from Amber to add flavour to the story, and I used a eulogy from Michelle Retterath to demonstrate how her friends felt.

Amber liked to educate and help people. I kept telling her as an adult that Emerson said that if you helped *one* person or changed their life, you were a success. Walt Whitman had a stroke when he was fifty-two years of age which left him severely disabled. A little more than ten years later, he wrote in his journal that he had come to terms with the disability which had made him feel "violently exiled from his own body." He wrote in his journal that he discovered that the most successful part of his life were his "ardent" friends and his loving relatives. I felt Amber had achieved that.

I hoped that my story about risk factors, precarious work, meaningful work, loneliness, criticism of the healthcare system, the lack of female research, medical gaslighting, and my experiences during and after Amber's death might help one person, change one person's attitude, and make Amber's experience more meaningful.

AMBER

Amber was our second child. Her sister, Molly, was twenty-three months older. My husband, Doug, and I met at university. Doug and I were pharmacists at one time, but we are retired now, and we were retired during Amber's journey. In a way, that was a blessing because we didn't have to worry about showing up to work during her hospitalization, nor did we have to worry about getting her to and from work. Looking back, the time we spent in the car with her was extra time that might have not happened if she had been living in Toronto. The time Amber spent curled up in bed each night playing video games with the dog between us, while her father sat in his chair in the same room, is now treasured time.

One day, long ago when she was young, I discovered Amber crying and found out that she was crying because her book was sad. I knew then, that she was hooked on reading. As a lifelong reader, she owned countless novels, and books on activism, feminism, art, civilization, and philosophy.

Amber went through the terrible twos and she didn't nap with a ride in the car like her sister had, so my husband found it a bit harder to get things done while I was working. One of my most cherished memories of Amber was when she was singing "Itsy Bitsy Spider" while sitting on my lap during a cruise up in Muskoka one summer. She sang herself to sleep all the time, and later on, as a teenager, she listened to music before bedtime. On my way home from work after picking the kids up at daycare, I often had to stop by the grocery store for milk or whatever. I have memories of Amber singing songs to me while sitting in the grocery cart. Little ditties that began with little rabbit "Frou Frou" and ended with the rabbit lopping all the heads off of the animals, or songs when the baby goes down the drain with bathwater. I would be shocked by the ending of the songs. I also remember dragging a screaming toddler out of the grocery store while one of my customers would say, "Oh, you have one too!"

Amber was a good student and she would have been able to take a science course or the fine art she chose at university. She added Philosophy to her major and graduated with distinction with a double major—Fine Art and Philosophy.

She also began FEAST with another student after graduating with a Masters of Fine Art from Ontario College of Art and Design University (OCADU). FEAST was a micro-funding dinner where you paid what you could afford, and people were encouraged to apply for funding for an art project that they envisioned. The proceeds from the dinner, above the costs, would be divided into grants for the artists. Projects were presented at the dinner, then the people voted on them. They held several dinners, funded several projects. This was the beginning of Amber's political and philanthropic life. It was through some of these projects, and articles I read in the magazine where she worked, that I realized how political art can be. I hadn't realized the importance of how art shaped people's thoughts. I appreciated art and creativity in my life, but its effect on others had not been in my thoughts. I did know that in the Middle Ages, art depicted Bible stories because most people could not read, so they learned the Bible stories through art. When Amber was going to take Fine Art, I didn't know that art criticized our culture and also influenced it.

AN ESSAY BY AMBER ABOUT GROWING UP

It Happened in the Woods

Come away, O human child!

To the waters and the wild

With a faery hand in hand

For the World is more

full of weeping

than you can understand.

—The Stolen Child, Will Yeats

I spent my childhood in a suburban world with large grassy backyards and quiet streets where children rode on bicycles and played catch in the road. I lived about a fifteen-minute walk from my grade school. Every day, on my walk to and from school[,] I would pass a small grove of trees. Living as I did amidst suburbia, that little grove of trees was like a wooded forest, dark and deep. There was no such phrase as old growth in my vocabulary. I would dawdle on my way home from school[,] exploring the creek that the trees hid from view, jumping from one side of the stream of water to the other. My little woods offered a place for the imagination to run wild, with twisting roots peeking their way out of the ground to trip up and trick you. As in fairy tales, it was easy to imagine that monsters hid in the woods of my childhood.

Suburbia only offers the illusion of safety, in the same way that my collection of trees offered the illusion of a forest. While I, with all the impetuousness of youth, imagined children-stealing goblins inhabiting the forest, around the corner from where I lived[,] a young woman was taken in the middle of the night off of her own front porch. The whispered rumour throughout the neighbourhood was that her parents—fed up with her tardiness at curfew—locked her out and went to bed, on the very night she forgot her keys, that night she was taken.

After that, I remember my parents developed tight, pinched looks of concern if I took too long walking home from school. That fifteen-minute walk that I had always stretched out to half an hour, or forty-five minutes—those stolen moments of youthful independence—took on a different meaning when compared to the very real experience of the missing girl. Of course, my experience of those events is clouded with the safe fear of a child—of still believing that there was no such thing as monsters that my parents couldn't soothe away. I was not quite old enough to understand that the real monsters in the world were not to be found in the woods. In all the stories I knew of children being kidnapped and taken away, there was always an element of the story that depicted the stolen child as better off, protected and suspended in youthful innocence where they would never have to learn about the real dangers that could be found in the world.

Patricia Beatty's installation, It Happened in the Woods, *conjures up the illusion of a forest. Beattie's stage, built through a combination of clay and trees, transforms the space into something both sinister and romantic. Beattie's forest should not be taken for the real thing, but rather[,] a complex set inviting the viewer to explore. If I close my eyes, I can imagine myself some place else, the forest of my childhood. Breathing in deeply[,] I find myself surrounded by the smell of the woods. The sound of water running through pipes becomes a trickling stream, the concrete floor feels like soft, rich earth, and the cracks in the floor become gnarled roots poking through the ground. The idea of walking through crooked pathways, unsure of whether the creaking branches are due to the wind or because of something more dangerous lurking in the shadows[,] gives me a delicious thrill that creeps up my spine. Of course, the deliciousness of the horror is tempered by the fact that there really is nothing to fear in these woods, no skulking dangers and no real monsters.*

Speaking to Beattie about the installation, she comments on this mixture of fear and play, describing the moment right before you start running because you are so scared, and how, in that moment, you find that you can't help laughing. It is that exhilaration that this installation is meant to invoke—the strength and overwhelming belief in your own safety. We laugh when we run away because always, at the back of our minds, most of all, we believe in our own ability to get away. In the woods[,] monsters aren't real, they are only as strong as we imagine them to be. The forests of our childhoods are romantic, dark[,] and deep. The trees envelope us[,] and we relax with the knowledge that sometimes[,] we are safer in the woods. (2011-2012)

This is Amber's version of what happened with Leslie Mahaffey, Kristen French, and Nina De Villiers. It is not exactly accurate, but she was a very young girl when this happened. The emotional effect is real. I thought that we had hid our anxiety better than we had. I really didn't want to have Amber know that I didn't sleep for months because of nightmares. I did not realize how much our worries had shown on our faces. I went through a sleepless time. I worried about finding the white car that had been described in the news. I worried about finding a body along the beach. Nina De Villiers was taken from a spot just a few city blocks from where we lived. We purchased an alarm system and had an emergency button that the kids could press. I suppose that really became an important happening in Amber's life. Her glade of trees is real, and I did not know that she was jumping the creek. Her imagination was always vivid.

DREAMS ARE FOR THE WEAK

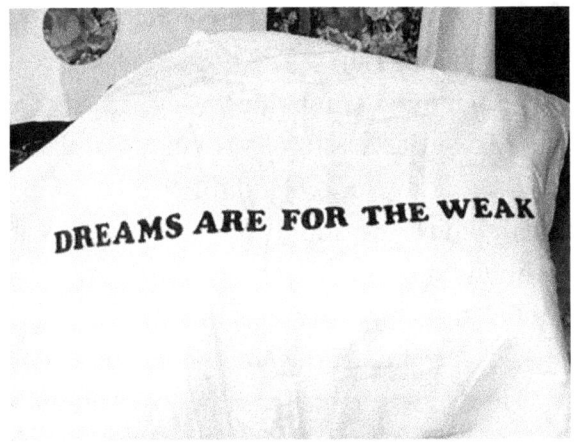

Amber did an art project at university called *Confessions*. Some of the confessions were on banners that flew from people's balconies or hung in Amber's apartment picture window. Some were on pillowcases like the one I have shown. I don't think they were necessarily Amber's own confessions, just statements that might be confessed by someone. I am not entirely sure why they were pillow cases that you slept on. Conceptual art is way over my head sometimes.

I don't believe Amber really thought dreams were for the weak. Amber had many dreams over the years. Some involved living in New York City, and some were for living on a farm with many pets.

She dreamed of living alone in an apartment somewhere, preferably Toronto or Guelph. She had always had to share because apartments were so expensive, and she longed for a place of her own. Toronto had the art scene and Guelph had a lot of university friends who had stayed in Guelph. She collected things for her new apartment. Casserole dishes, coffee makers, coffee bean grinders, cookbooks, and a Dutch oven. The recipe books were eclectic, including ethnic cooking. When she had energy, she would try recipes that I wouldn't cook or eat. I am your basic meat and potatoes, with the occasional rice dish or pasta. Amber began cooking and taking the food for lunches at work. We sometimes searched high and low for odd spices like sumac that aren't stocked in the average grocery store of a small city. Eventually, she started ordering them online. What would we do without online shopping?

Amber had a favourite dream of working in a place where dogs were allowed to come to work. She did her internship at one such place and talked almost incessantly about the dog. She befriended the neighbourhood cats in one place that she lived.

Amber wanted to take pottery lessons but her schedule at the store she worked at wouldn't accommodate for that. She was so disappointed. She also wanted to learn how to sew, and specifically, quilt. She became a fabric collector. I made some quilts as baby gifts and wedding gifts for her friends. I helped her mark the fabric for a quilt that she chose to learn which was completely made of the flying geese block. The flying geese have triangles in the oblongs and you must try to make them so you don't cut off the tips of the triangles when you sew them together. Not the easiest pattern for a beginner. After she died, I finished the quilt. She had chosen all the colours. Her friend thought that the geese looked like the back of envelopes and thought the quilt was full of love letters from Amber. I gave her the quilt. How could I not when she had described it so wonderfully?

Amber still dreamt of finding the perfect job, or at least one that challenged her, had reasonable hours so she could see her friends, and paid a living wage.

When Amber was growing up, she often had stones in her pocket or knapsack. They were beautiful to her, but often, I thought of them as ordinary. I think Amber dreamt of pretty stones in her life and she became a rock/crystal/mineral collector. She had big pieces of rose quartz, agate, and geodes that had been split into two, showing a beautiful design within. Many of the stones were given to a friend at her request, but later, I found a few that were packed away in separate boxes. I have a glass vase almost filled with small stones of various types. Amber believed in healing by crystals. She had a book about crystals and their healing properties too. I think Amber dreamt that life could be magical, and therefore, crystals could heal our wounds.

Amber also dreamt of work for everyone that was equitable and paid such that you weren't part of the working poor. She came to us with the theory of Universal Basic Income for everyone. We thought the idea would never take foothold. We thought it was pie in the sky thinking. But Amber explained that this concept had been tried and tested in various communities before and had been more successful than was expected. The Basic Income helped people start businesses or return to school to obtain better jobs, and these people added to the community. Later, it actually became a trial in some communities in Ontario, and I was already educated about it by Amber. The Conservatives did stop the study way before they could measure any outcomes.

At no time would I ever entertain that Amber was weak for dreaming. She read books about labour movements that began with doughnuts, for example. She was adamant that life could be made better for everyone. Her dreams were plentiful, what some would say *a field of dreams*.

One of the dreams that came true was a trip to Greece, Turkey, and Israel. I was never sure why that trip caught her eleven-year-old fancy. I just saw her head pop up while the Priest described it. She was excited by the travel and the trip. Doug and I considered it and thought it could be beneficial as a learning experience for both children, and we took our savings for their post-secondary learning and invested in this unusual trip. I think we all learned a lot of history, and even some mythology. The trip was inspiring. Those experiences were used over and over again by the kids. I found the trip memorable. Amber loved to travel and became very capable with the camera. With photography lessons in high school, she looked at courses in university that would accommodate or use the camera.

When the high school had a trip to Italy and France, she went out and found a job to fund the trip, and she had a very memorable time on that European adventure. One of her friends hired a limo, and the girls left for the airport in style. They were all excited. There were other trips after that, and each one developed her skills as a photographer and her knowledge of art history.

SOME OF AMBER'S ART

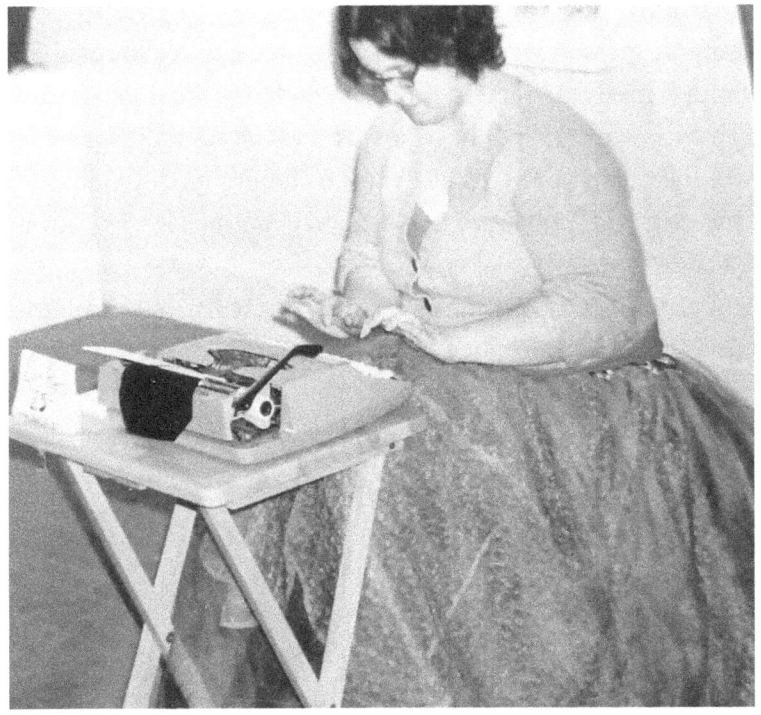

One project of Amber's evolved as she tried different venues for it. This picture is for one of her first performances. For a quarter, she would write a poem for you, on a subject of your choosing. The typewriter was like the ones my sister had when I was in high school, long ago in the early seventies. This typewriter had no ribbon though, so you could not see the poem until the end when she removed the copy from behind the carbon paper. I was surprised she could find carbon paper in this day and age. When I was in university, we all carried carbon paper so that we could take notes for someone who was absent, or in my case, for when I fell asleep in the middle of class. I do not completely understand the whole concept of the poetry project. Part of the concept was that she was giving part of her work, her thoughts, herself, for a very small price. She wanted to make peoples' lives better any way she could. In San Diego, she performed the poetry again, but this time the cost of the poem was anything the person was willing to give. She got slips for paid fines at the library, used bus tickets, a broken watch, a toothbrush, a coffee card that may or may not have any coffees left on it. She never had a copy of the poem because there was no ribbon in the typewriter. She had the title of the poem on a plastic bag, and what was paid inside the bag.

Amber wrote all the time as a child. She wrote letters of apology to me, cards that said she loved me, and very interesting stories and poems. She wrote for magazines when she was older, and also introductions into books. Some of her art pieces revolved around words—she played with them in art. Her Philosophy major was language-focused.

AMBER AND HEROES

Our society has not changed, and neither have the themes of our stories. The power of one person is often examined. The Ancient Greeks had superheroes who were gods, or humans with half of their DNA inherited from gods. Many of the heroes were hyper-masculine men, and there were very few women portrayed as heroes. Women have been taught the role of the damsel in distress. Female heroes created by women use cleverness, curiosity, and determination to accomplish their work. They are also more intelligent and less brutal than the male heroes.

Heroes are important to society because they consummate a wish-fulfillment fantasy. We unconsciously feel that if we had super-human strength. It is also felt by some that heroes expand our idea of possibility. Our existence has been described as "lives of quiet desperation," and this may be because our thoughts of possibility are too small. Hero stories renew our hope, and that is why we never get bored with the many variations of the familiar hero story. Everyone, at some time, needs to be rescued, and heroes give temporary relief. Superheroes represent a standard to strive for and they are ideal role models. Our favorite heroes are chosen by our ideals, and what the hero represents. Our hero choices are symbols of what we would like to possess, and the ambitions we would like to satisfy. Yet, today's youth mix up celebrity with heroism, and often choose an athlete, musician, or movie star to represent their personal hero, or they use the fictional heroes of Spiderman and Superman. One of Amber's favourite heroes at the time of her illness was Ruth Bader Ginsberg. Personal heroes from real life can be an issue because they probably have weaknesses and character flaws. After all, they are human. This makes them more like us, but it doesn't negate the good they have performed.

In university, one of Amber's projects explored superheroes. Amber had dressed in a long pink prom dress with gloves up over the elbows and a pink updo wig, and she tried to change in a phone booth, which was pretty tricky. Amber felt that superheroes had the quotidian mundane tasks of living as well as we mere humans. She tried taking the bus, her friend filmed it all, and she got in trouble for using the ATM dressed like that. Every hero needed to get cash. Laundry needs to accomplished, so Amber tried that at the laundromat, from which she was kicked out. Groceries are also needed by the superhero, so she tried to do her purchasing in her costume, and the grocery store was not happy. So, all in all, misunderstood. Futility and failure as a learning experience were often among Amber's themes in her art. Through her art work and studies, she realized that it was okay to fail—something her mother didn't learn. In failing, you learned what did work and what didn't. I don't think she was cynical in her exploration of the female hero. Perhaps, she was making a statement that as a female, there were also mundane chores expected to be done, or that we should be able to have a little whimsey in our lives by wearing outlandish costumes while doing mundane chores. I really think it was the camera that was the issue.

Superheroes are usually dedicated in fighting the evil of the universe. Some think that superheroes being introduced to children helps them learn about courage, self-sacrifice, self-control, and willpower. Some feel the popularity of the anti-hero introduces human characteristics and weaknesses to us. Sometimes they do something right, even when the method is legally wrong, and they do it without apology. The anti-hero is becoming more acceptable in today's world, but it may be making our ethics questionable.

Saving the world was paramount to Amber. She never gave up trying. Amber liked hero stories as much as I did. Saving the day, winning, and solving mysteries, but the ladies are smart, capable, and break a lot of rules. The men they are with support and keep them whole as the women launch out to destroy evil. David and Goliath stories and themes can be found in many books and films. Even while on her death bed, Amber was trying to save the world in her drug or disease-induced hallucinations, and she had me there as a back-up.

AMBER AT WORK

Amber started working at a coffee and donut shop in high school to help finance a school trip to Italy. After that, she moved on to a drugstore. Amber was given more responsibility as her experience increased from cashier supervisor to assistant store manager, until she became an office manager for an alternative therapy clinic. Amber decided to return to school for her Master of Fine Arts.

While doing her Master's program, she worked as a teaching assistant. Part of her coursework at OCADU required a student internship. Most internships were unpaid. She began work at an art magazine, learned editing design, and wrote for them. Generally, she could put the whole magazine together and voluntarily kept on in the internship for almost two years, as well as doing her other school work. It was a bit upsetting for us because it was unpaid and prevented her from getting a paid job. She needed help with rent and groceries. When the editor position became available, she interviewed for the job. She was very disappointed because someone else got it, and this disillusioned Amber. She had poured her heart and soul into the unpaid position and she could do all the jobs required on the magazine.

After that, Amber became a vocal proponent of paid internships. She told her students not to work for free and she joined *The Precarious Workers Brigade*, writing articles and doing interviews about internships. This group is part of the *Carrot Workers' Collective* and is based in the U.K. Internships were, historically, paid positions, until labour was weakened by the Thatcher/Reagan governments.

Still, the people working there are very committed and willing to go into debt, thinking of it as a route to a later job in that company.

Amber did work as a part-time instructor for night courses at OCADU for two semesters, but that was the upper limit for a contract for a part-time person to be employed there. Jobs in arts and teaching at the college level are precarious. This was something Amber faced, and a primary reason for the depression she developed later in her job experience.

Amber was finally offered a job in her field as a director of an art gallery run by the student union, *XPACE*. Unfortunately, this was also a contract position. Amber was able to have her contract renewed for another term and a half because she was relocating the gallery. While in the position, she negotiated benefits for the three employees, including herself and the intern. She felt it was meaningful work. After the contract, Amber could not find another job in her field. She interviewed well, but there was always someone with more experience.

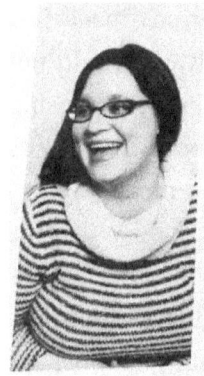

AMBER LANDGRAFF

Amber is an artist/curator who uses community and political engagement as an integral part of her curatorial and artistic practice. She has an MFA in Criticism and Curatorial Practices, and has facilitated, and collaborated on such events as Building Together, FEAST Toronto and Toronto Free Gallery's The Bridge series. She is currently the director at XPACE Cultural Centre, a not-for-profit artist run centre that focuses on supporting and offering professional opportunities to student and emerging artists.

amber@xpace.info

Sometimes, I thought Amber was overreaching, pursuing jobs she *could* do but did not have the job *experience* for. Employers are not willing to train the staff anymore. They want you to hit the ground running. I think this is very short-sighted, but that is how it is today. Amber was a bright, eager-to-learn, conscientious woman who was capable of work that was challenging. She longed for meaningful work.

As her mother, I was biased, of course, but I also knew her potential was not being reached or used in the job. It was very hard to watch someone being frustrated by a system that is not willing to train and nurture young people. She was underutilized in many of her jobs. I cheered for her when she was interviewing and trying for new jobs and was just as sad when the offers of employment were given elsewhere. Or limited by arbitrary rules. Life can be an emotional rollercoaster and as mothers, we also feel our children's despair. Jane Jacobs, in *Dark Age Ahead*, spoke of the constant rejection of the unemployed and "the quiet despair that the world had no place for them," (2005).

After her employment insurance and odd jobs of editing or writing ran out, Amber had to move home. We had downsized in the interim to a smaller house and lacked room for her belongings. We paid for the movers and the storage.

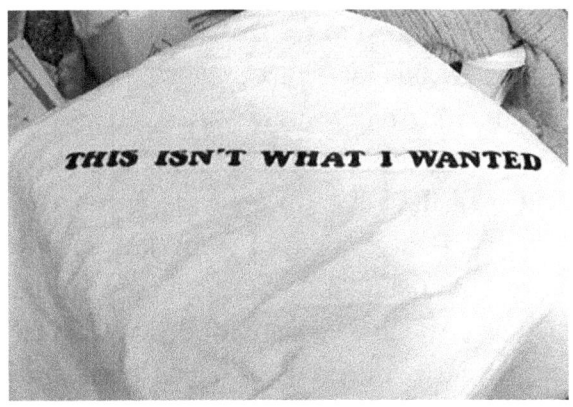

When Amber moved in with us, she found a part-time casual job at a retail establishment. She was guaranteed twenty-five hours a week. She was also placed at a store about half hour's drive from Barrie. Amber didn't have her driver's license so we had to deliver her there and then return to pick her up. Jobs within the company that were in her toolbox of experience were not available because she was not full-time. She had been a cashier and cashier supervisor since she was in her teens, so the job did not give her a sense of purpose or any chance of promotion, but she needed the funds and this one was what was available. She could not find peace and fulfillment from this type of job, a job that she had been doing in high school and university. Amber could not "settle into her job and enjoy it" for what it was, a job. This job, and the difficulties with it, were part of the reason that Amber became so isolated from her friends. She was lonely and I learned later that these things were important because they were risk factors in her health. The advantages of full-time were benefits, with two days off each week. Unfortunately, Amber had no control of her shifts. If she was scheduled, she had to work, often ninety consecutive days stretches with no time off. We were obliged to drive her. It severely hampered Amber's social life, as well as our own. It exhausted her. She couldn't have friends to visit and she couldn't visit Toronto because her evening and weekend shifts were difficult to plan around. I know firsthand what it is like to work evenings and weekends, which I did most of my career. It is hard to see friends when they work Monday to Friday, and the friends just don't understand how different your schedule is than theirs. Amber was living to work instead of working to live. These feelings of being owned by corporations are not unusual. In fact, Copaken felt these issues were widespread, and even white-collar workers felt this, every hour of every day. Isolation came with the constant working required (2021). The employer gives nothing with security, but demands all your loyalty, your total availability, according to their need. It is toxic capitalism. Stiglitz, an economist, wrote that capitalism as we know it is "delivering inequality, pollution, unemployment, and most of all, the degradation of values to the point where everything is acceptable, and no one is accountable," (quoted in Maté, 2022). Chomsky said that "democratic freedom and free will rarely stray from what is socially acceptable, even if it is a threat to our species," (quoted in Maté, 2022). Our acceptance in society is only conditionally awarded to those who follow the system.

Betrayal by corporations was discussed by James Hollis as a "betrayal of our hope that the world might be manageable and predictable. As we grow older, we find repeated affronts to our sense of self, our capacity to control the outcome," (2005). I think this describes Amber's experience very well.

In his autobiography, *The Seven Storey Mountain*, Thomas Merton argued that we mistakenly believe perfection relies on the thoughts, opinions, and applause of others. This belief leads us to feel real only when we exist in others imagination. According to Erich Fromm, society focuses on meeting expectations, rather than what is genuinely good for people. With advertising and peer pressure, Merton also observed that society tries to "excite every nerve in the human body and keep it at the highest pitch of artificial tension" in order to sell us more things and more remedies. We to try and cope, but the constant excitation wears out our bodies, and the constant tension makes us feel valueless. In attempts to alleviate our anxiety and dissatisfaction, we purchase things. It becomes an addictive cycle. The anxiety and purchasing distracts us "from real needs, real emotions, and real life," (Maté, 2022)

Pre-COVID loneliness was a major theme in *The American Psychological Association's Journal* in 2015. I knew that loneliness accentuated depression, but I was not aware that it posed a health risk comparable to smoking fifteen cigarettes per day and was associated with a twenty- six percent increase in mortality (Maté, 2022). It can also be comparable to the risks of alcohol abuse. Loneliness can present a health risk equivalent or greater to obesity and can break your DNA strands. Loneliness has been found to increase inflammation within the body which could limit your mobility, inhibit the immune system, making you more apt to be sick with colds and flu, and decrease the effectiveness of killer cells to stop cancer cells in your body. It can also increase the risk of cardiovascular disease, leading to strokes and death. Social isolation was found by Umberson and Karas Montez to result in "psychological and physical disintegration and even death," (2011). The mobility issues and depression can further increase your social isolation. Loneliness has also been linked to burnout. This enhanced the importance of Amber's need for days off, it potentially affected Amber's health, and ultimately, perhaps, her cancer. Amber suffered from many colds and tonsilitis. I did know she was lonely and was frustrated by her schedule. The scheduler seemed to forget that there were people's lives in that schedule. I was equally frustrated because I had worked retail most of my life, and we had never treated people so poorly. We even arranged for Amber to see a counsellor to deal with the feelings she had developed during her working life. Loneliness was definitely a risk factor for her illness.

Amber had written about and curated shows about the insecurity and underutilization of employees in their workplace. She was caught up in the web she had tried to fight against. This is an explanation of an art installation about gig jobs that Amber had previously written when she was still at the art gallery:

"We may find ourselves and our labouring bodies taken advantage of, the exploited and underrepresented. Precarity encourages a particular kind of vulnerability, and yet, for many workers, the instability and uncertainty that comes with a precarious work environment is an ongoing way of life. Young workers, those who work in the service industry, women, and people of color often find themselves in positions where their emotional labour is held hostage in exchange for a working environment that marginalizes, exploits, or makes invisible the work of their bodies. These days, it seems, it is not enough for us to do a job well, we also have to love doing it, or at least perform a convincing semblance of that love. Where are the moments for relief? Hourly wages make the hours spent performing a job significant, and even in situations where there might not be enough work to do, constant occupation is expected. A productive worker is one who can account for every moment of their time. However, when there isn't enough work to go around, that occupation becomes less productive, the worker must make ongoing attempts to find anything to do at all. Occupation again becomes a form of performance, as one cannot afford to admit that they don't have any meaningful work to do when they are shift workers and are paid by the hour.

*The performance is exhausting, and often doesn't end with the end of the workday. A lack of long-term stability means that we are constantly searching for work, and searching for the experiences that will make us competitive prospects for a limited number of jobs. We are a workforce that in many ways, never stops working . . . The final work of the show is a collaborative piece made by Spadafora and Enkel. One of the first things seen when entering the space is a giant denim work-shirt with a patch that reads, "**When this shift ends.**" Relief Support asks us to think about the time we spend working, the kind of work that we perform, and whether there are alternative ways for us to work together. Enkel and Spadafora's statement, "**When this shift ends**" is a significant one for a precarious workforce that never stops working. When this shift ends, I will take some time for myself, experience relief," (Landgraff, 2015).*

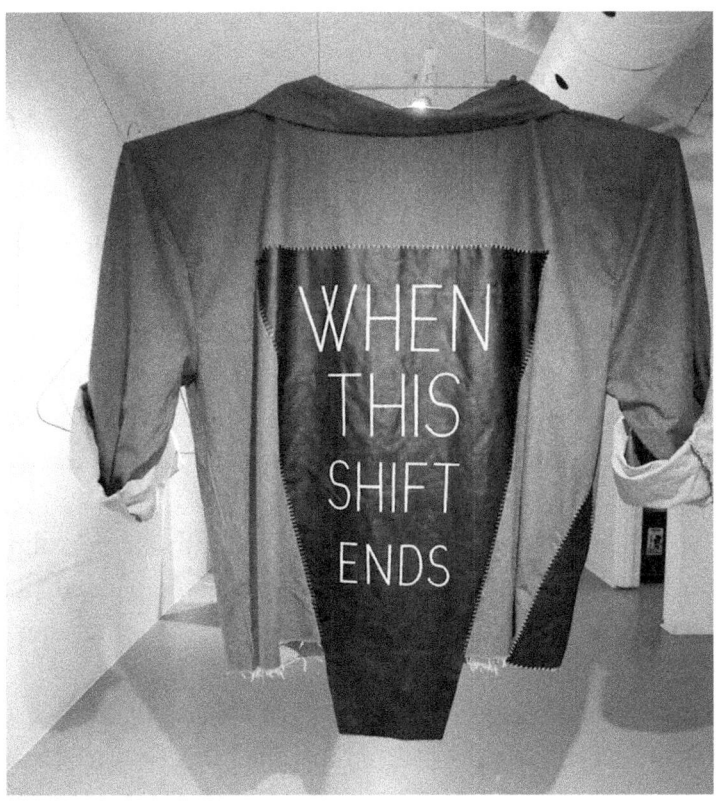

Work as a "depleting, dispirited experience," was found to be common by Maté, a traumatist and addiction treatment physician, and he felt it was getting worse (2022). A GALLUP poll across 142 countries found that only thirteen percent of people felt engaged at work. We all want meaning in our jobs, and Amber did not feel her job was meaningful. At the gallery, she taught people how to write resumes. She wrote resumes for others, posted all job or art opportunities on her social media, curated art shows, hosted them, and taught interns. The people she helped had their confidence boosted by the new resumes. Now, she was a cashier/stock person, a job she had been doing since her teens. It was hard to accept the drastic change in her job responsibilities. "Meaning is not found by the individual accomplishing their private goals, but with the core needs of belonging, relatedness, connectedness, autonomy, mastery, or competence," (Maté, 2022). Lack of meaning is not dependent on the valuation of others or achievement. It is knowing yourself to be part of something bigger than yourself. This definition of oneself is more about what one is *not*, rather than what one *is*, but we often define ourselves by what our job is. If there is meaning, many things can be made more endurable. Some people make up for a lack of meaning in their job by finding meaning in their spare time, but Amber had no extra time, or when she got the occasional day off, she was too exhausted to do anything else. She did become the union representative for her store and went to union meetings where she acted as secretary. She did bring coffee to striking teachers at Georgian College to show her solidarity.

In *Memories, Dreams, Reflections*, Jung felt that one's fullness of life was inhibited by meaninglessness, and he concluded that fact made it equivalent to illness. Lack or loss of meaning affects our health and nervous systems (Maté, 2022).

Chronic Stress, especially stress experienced daily like Amber was feeling, has been shown to inhibit the body's ability to destroy diseased cells throughout the body. Copaken said there were numerous studies showing "a causal effect between stress and the production of numerous growth factors that can actually speed the development of cancer," (2021). Stress, per se, does not *cause* cancer but *promotes* the conditions for increased tumor growth and spread (Maté, 2022). Potentially, the body contains cancer cells all the time, but the immune response fights them. Stress can alter the immune response. The inflammation from stress can also damage our DNA and affect the repair of the DNA, and it can also stimulate the blood vessels to bring more nutrients to the cancer cells.

The absence or the threatened loss of something, whether the loss is "the loss of love, work, dignity, self-esteem, or meaning," creates stress. The body perceives the loss as necessary for survival (Maté,2022). Long-term stress can deplete levels of cortisol, and this depletion becomes a marker for burnout or a predictor for future disease. In Canada, it was found that if women were under economic pressure while pregnant, afterwards, the child, by the age of six, may have increased cortisol and this increases the risk of disease. As a pharmacist, my job was very stressful and time crunched. Did working under those conditions increase the cortisol levels in my children?

The stress, loneliness, and lack of meaning affected many body systems and possibly contributed to the cancer Amber developed. Her constant short-term jobs and searching for a place to belong also affected her mental health. I guess it acts as a warning to pursue jobs that were healthier. Yet, that is exactly what Amber did— she searched.

The social macrocosm manifests as illness, Maté said, and the social roles and characteristics we are taught have a cumulative effect on our health. We live in a patriarchal society where women are often given the role of caregiver. This role is never finished at the end of the day. Women are expected to be socially acceptable, suppress their anger, and be the emotional glue holding the nuclear family, extended family, and community together (2022). Women act as glue, but the glue holding our bodies together (connective tissue) gets attacked by diseases such as Lupus, Scleroderma, Fibromyalgia, and Rheumatoid Arthritis because of the stress of our emotional labour. The body's integrity is eroded, and the ability to survive is decreased. Yet, women are taught by society to ignore the signals and put others first. Fibromyalgia has been the bane of my life, causing me to become disabled in 2000. Amber had seen a pain specialist about her chronic pain being possible fibromyalgia after she had been working for a bit, probably in her late twenties. The pain specialist pooh-poohed the idea and said fibromyalgia was psychological, and a learned behavior. This phenomenon has been called medical gaslighting and is the subject in many articles and books recently. He embarrassed and angered Amber. Her pain was real and she felt undermined. The corollary was that he implied my illness was not real either, and this was not lost on Amber. He negated the real pain she was feeling. Multiple Sclerosis, another disease that had been gaslighted by medicine, was also thought to be psychological until the late sixties. I think medical gaslighting was also present later in Amber's story.

Pain cannot be seen by a doctor. He may see the grimace that implies pain, and a certain tension in the body, but he cannot see it, so it is difficult for the doctor to believe someone is really in pain. Migraine headaches are also often negated. Pain that women experience, and the phenomenon of ignoring women's pain by misogynist doctors, is starting to get much more attention these days.

It has been found that women develop chronic diseases long before old age. They have twice the number of cases of anxiety and depression and are more at risk for autoimmune disease. Consequently, they spend more years with poor health and disability than the average man. They may have a larger *quantity* of life, but the *quality* is less than men (Maté, 2022).

AMBER'S JOURNEY
The Beginning: May 2018

*"Women's anger needs to be honoured and celebrated and protected—
the way virginity used to be. Female Anger is a discipline, a repertory
of styles. Each requires vocal, gestural, emotional skills; a clear sense
of what the situation offers and how the story unfolds. Growing girls
need anger models, muses, coaches, and exemplars."*

—Margo Jefferson

I don't know when the illness started. I think it had been brewing for
a long time before any of the severe symptoms showed up. Near the
end of April, Amber began to bleed vaginally—an abnormally excessive amount. It was nothing like she had ever experienced. She also
had a lot of lower back pain, which should have been taken more
seriously by the doctors who saw her. Her constant companion was
pain and the heating pad, until it burnt out and we had to buy a
new one.

The bleeding was so heavy that it went through a sanitary pad, her
clothes, and the cushion on the dining room chair. She was appalled
and embarrassed. We took her to the Emergency Department (ED)
and waited the usual four to six hours. Amber was prescribed a drug
to stop the bleeding or make it more livable. This trip was made
again later that week, and more of the drug was given.

By the middle of May, Amber was starting to gasp for breath and
vomiting, as well as still bleeding. When we complained about her

breathing, the family physician wanted more lab work done, and we were sent by the family doctor to the ED again.

Unfortunately, Amber answered that the bleeding was primarily wrong instead of saying the breathing was that day's issue. It was true the odyssey began with bleeding, but she was struggling for breath. I am surprised the nurses didn't notice it. The nurse took blood, but they weren't the tests we needed, and they also did a pregnancy test for the third time! The wait time when we entered the ED was estimated by the computer to be about three hours, but then two accidents came in and a heart attack, and the wait time climbed to six hours. There is no privacy in the waiting room. You learn things you would rather not know, or shouldn't know. You see things that entertain you during the long wait. The ED has since changed how it works, and psychiatric patients are sent to a different area. We waited six hours until Amber was finally shown a bed, so I searched for food. I thought a fruit smoothie might appeal to Amber and stay down better than food, so I got that, and a sandwich for me. When I arrived back, the doctor had just arrived. He had a harried morning and didn't hear about breathing issues (or might not have *allowed* us to tell him about the breathing issues and blood work the family doctor wanted). He had an attitude! Bleeding? How *dare* we come to the Emergency Department with *vaginal bleeding*? Didn't we know that it was normal for many women to bleed that much, and Amber should accept it as a fact of life and expect it *for the rest of her life*? Amber's face went white with shock, and you could see the dismay that this might be the rest of her life. I was angry. I wondered if I had gone to sleep, and awakened in the nineteenth century. I told him this was *not* normal, primarily since it differed from her previous history. Women should not have to live like that, and did he not realize what *a life sentence* he had just cursed her with? He *hadn't examined her* or asked any questions. I couldn't believe that Amber was being ignored. Did he still believe that women were born to be in pain and that it was just hysterics? I asked for a gynecology consult at the very least. I forgot about the breathing issue because I was so angry. He agreed to write a consult, and that was the second request for a gynecological consult she received. The first consultation we asked for was at the beginning of May and we were still waiting. Later, we learned that our city was experiencing a severe shortage of gynecologists.

Amber and I felt embarrassed and humiliated by the physician. Bessie Van der Kolk, a Traumatologist, was quoted in Maté, that "we are traumatized when we are not seen," (2022). In 2017, the U.K.'s All-Party Parliamentary Group on Women's Health found that "women were not treated with dignity," not given enough information about their illness or health, and no data was collected for study (Jackson, 2021). We were afraid to go to the ED again even though the vomiting and breathlessness increased, she was in a lot of pain, and she was not eating.

Gabrielle Jackson wrote that "there are still physicians who don't believe it is their job to listen to women" and believe that "women's natural state is to be in pain," (2021). Although the pain might not be killing us normally, "it is denying our full humanity," and opportunities are lost because physicians refuse to understand the facts of life in women's lives, and this situation doesn't have to be the answer. This is what medical gaslighting is about.

There are several factors why doctors may ignore women. Rebecca Puhl found that dismissal of patients' symptoms shows that the combined effects of sexism and weight bias are clear (2011). Physicians have not received enough training, the research is missing, they don't know the answer, they are working within a system that makes it hostile to treat women with complex problems because of *time* restraints within the system, and society is still largely patriarchal. Only a few minutes is allowed for a doctor to see a patient. It really is like an assembly line in a car factory, but with more at stake. Jackson felt that most doctors wanted to help, but culture and medicine are still sexist. Budgets still exist that restrict the length of time that can be spent with each patient (Jackson, 2021).

Dusenbery also wrote about medicine needing to catch up with research information into the female reproductive system (2017). A marketing study conducted in 2016, "The Eve Appeal," interviewed one thousand women across the U.K. It found almost twenty percent of women would not report abnormal bleeding to their doctor. Women are still embarrassed to speak about their reproductive organs to the doctor. For a long time, women have been taught that it is taboo to talk about their problems, especially reproductive ones, yet women must talk about their cycle confidently if we want better care. It was also discovered that many women don't know the proper names of their anatomy and don't understand their own bodies (Jackson, 2021). Jackson pointed out that "one reason for diagnostic delay is women, like their doctor, thought their painful periods were normal, and did not ask about them." Despite the women's movement and the realization in the 1980s that there was little research on women's health, things haven't changed much in 2018, or 2023 for that matter. I found this information to be very disappointing.

Although the U.S. government has asked for women's research since 1993, as I write this in 2024, not much had advanced. In February 2024, Lady Biden announced one hundred million dollars in funding to women's health. Vice President Kamala Harris said women's reproductive health had been in crisis since Roe vs. Wade was overturned in 2022. The need for research on women's health has now become news in 2024.

I was surprised when I read these books five years after Amber's experience. I went to university during the feminist movement in the 1970s and studied a health profession (Pharmacy). We studied the pharmacology of birth control pills and they knew where in the reproductive cycle they acted. This may have been the drug companies that did the research, but I assumed that much was known. I suppose the problems with the research were that the diseases of the reproductive system were not studied. Were we that far behind? I did not understand the cost of endometriosis on women's lives until I read these books. I guess we are behind.

Does society teach females that they are meant to suffer? Dusenbury felt it did. I had never considered this, nor questioned my belief system, yet I had experienced these things myself. I suffered for more than thirty years with the pain from my reproductive system. How accepting we are about society's impact! Like Abby Norman, "I trusted that doctors knew how to fix people—so long as they wanted to be fixed," (2018). There are so many things that medicine cannot fix, and I was aware of this. I didn't realize they knew so little about the female reproductive system, and women's pain seems as though they were not worthy of study, yet, we can fix some genetic diseases with cutting the DNA. I, like Dusenbery, "had expected to be taken seriously." I took for granted my new equality in society, yet struggled "with policies, institutions, and norms that have not changed as much as our expectations," (2018).

BREATHING: JUNE 2018

"Breath is intrinsically full of grace."

I had noticed Amber gasping for breath, and it was more severe by mid-June. I was concerned, but Amber assured me she had phoned the doctor who had ordered *Symbicort* to help her breathe. It opens the passageways in the lungs and relieves inflammation. It did not help, and I asked Amber to call the doctor again. Amber was frustrated with the breathlessness and with me, but did not keep calling the doctor like I would have. I think she just doubted herself, and she accepted the lack of help. I, on the other hand, was not accepting this for her and I called the doctor myself. After seeing the doctor in the office, Amber was once again advised to go to the ED. Once again, we sat in the waiting room for the five or six hours wait and finally entered the ED, where we waited for a CT scan, and then waited for the scan to be read. From where I sat, I could see the nurse's station, and men who were not the nurses were gathered around a computer screen puzzling at what was shown. Part of me knew this was Amber's scan. Eventually, the doctor came in and said the respiratory specialist was coming. When he arrived, the specialist told us he thought Amber had Sarcoidosis. I asked if Sarcoidosis also affected the reproductive organs, and he didn't answer. It always blew my mind that they tested Amber for pregnancy every time and then ushered Doug and I out of the room to ask her if she might be pregnant. Amber was not a young teenager; she was an adult and we understood this. She had been bleeding heavily for more than six weeks. How could she be pregnant? I was somewhat relieved that there was finally a partial diagnosis. Some progress was made. The nurse told us that Amber needed to be admitted. She was given oxygen. Amber and her friends were skeptical of the diagnosis. They all knew that if Sarcoidosis was the potential diagnosis on the medical program *HOUSE*, it was *never* Sarcoidosis.

Sarcoidosis is an autoimmune disease. For some reason, the immune system starts to fail. Tiny grain-like clusters of inflamed cells called granulomas form most commonly (in nearly ninety percent of cases) in the lung and lymph nodes of the armpit or groin. Signs and symptoms depend on the location of the granulomas, but they include fatigue, swollen lymph nodes, weight loss, pain and swelling in the joints, persistent cough, shortness of breath, and wheezing. Chest pain can be present if the granulomas are in the lungs. It can also be in the brain, presenting as skin rashes or nodules under the skin. It can also affect the heart. I could not find anything about vaginal bleeding or pelvic pain when I googled. I think the physician was in love with the diagnosis of Sarcoidosis. They admitted Amber that night. Amber got some pain medication and a steroid, and was still on oxygen. The next day was Saturday, and not much happens in the way of tests on the weekend in a hospital. I think it was on Saturday that we were told that there was a granuloma in Amber's brain. That threw me. The brain! My brilliant daughter with something in her brain! The specialist assured us that it could happen with Sarcoidosis and could go away with treatment. Again, I asked about the bleeding, and he told me that wasn't his specialty. I asked for a gynecologist to look at Amber while she was in the hospital. That is the third time, from a third doctor, that I had requested a gynecologist.

On Sunday, they decided that a blind biopsy would be performed in the ICU since the operating rooms were closed, and guided biopsies only were done in Newmarket. Doug and I arrived at the ICU when instructed, and we were ushered into a waiting room and waited a long time. Finally, we were allowed to see Amber. The respirologist seemed flustered and asked why we hadn't said that Amber had sleep apnea. We said that question had never been explored by any doctor and there wasn't an official diagnosis. We suspected she had apnea, but Amber didn't believe us. Nothing had been done to investigate it. He didn't say as much but implied that they had encountered a big problem with the apnea while executing the biopsy. I think he had been frightened. It was a feeling deep in my soul.

The procedure which was done was when a physician blindly takes a sample and hopes that he gets the area that is problematic. It is a procedure in which if a negative result is obtained could be a false negative because they just didn't get the right area. I was skeptical of the purpose of that kind of biopsy, and after the trouble, I wondered why they even tried.

Amber remained in the hospital on oxygen and pain medication. A course of steroids was administered for a week. She was discharged because of the July first holiday. She was prescribed prednisone (a steroid), but *no oxygen or pain medication*. She was *not* seen by a gynecologist while in hospital.

DO NOT RESUSCITATE

On the first morning of Amber's hospitalization, the patient in the third bed of the ward had a cardiac arrest. The people responding to the arrest, the doctor specifically, were angry that she did not have a DNR (do not resuscitate) order. I had been in many family meetings when I had worked on a geriatric floor in another hospital and heard the ward doctor explain to the senior's family that resuscitating was painful, patients ended up with broken ribs, and often, the elderly died anyway. It was one of the first things addressed with the family on that floor. The doctor answering the code blue that day explained this to the patient, who agreed that resuscitation was not what she wanted. She wanted a DNR. She had been in the hospital for at least six weeks, most of that time in the ICU. Her lungs would fill up with fluid and needed draining several times daily. The doctor was amazed that this had not been addressed yet.

Amber was wide-eyed when we arrived that morning because she had witnessed the whole episode. She had only seen this done on television before. Shortly after we arrived, the woman's daughter appeared, creating chaos in the room. The daughter accused the staff of bullying her mother and asked how dare they put a DNR on her without her husband's permission. What they didn't realize was that if the patient was of sound mind, she was the one that gives permission, despite what the daughter and husband think. It is her body and her care. The poor nurses, they tried to explain, but nothing would calm the daughter and she left, saying it wasn't the end of the issue. The husband later arrived with the daughter, and more chaos ensued. A doctor and a social worker were paged, and the family would not calm down. The family threatened to go to the TV station and report that their mother was mistreated. The husband became more incensed and pulled out his health card and asked what it said on the card. It said "*health*," he said, and unless his wife walked out of the hospital in *perfect health*, everyone working there had failed in their job.

We all still have the fantasy of returning to our previous life at the risk of a prolonged, terrible death. In *The Death of Ivan Ilyich*, Tolstoy wrote that Ivan thought he would not die if he lay very still and took the remedy, and his health would return. Medicine has not improved that much since that novel was written. The reality of the disease is seldom discussed. Perhaps, the physicians are as delusional as we are (Gawende, 2019).

Security was called, and the family was escorted from the room. I know this was private, but it wasn't held privately. I kept wondering why the family wasn't escorted to a meeting room. It seemed cruel to be questioning this in front of the woman herself. The woman was still deemed capable of making her own decisions, yet there was not a peep from her. The staff tried to get the family into another room in the afternoon when the whole issue was debated again, but they wouldn't leave the ward. For that encounter, we asked if it was possible to remove Amber from the room while it was happening. She was put in a chair with oxygen that could travel with us and was pushed down to the sunroom.

Paul Kalanithi pondered his job as a physician in his book *When Breath Becomes Air*, which he wrote while dying from lung cancer: "The physician's duty is not to stave off death or return patients to their old lives, but to take into our arms the patient and family whose lives have disintegrated, and work until they can stand back up and face, make sense of, and own existence," (2016).

This incident led to a long discussion with Amber about what had happened in the room, and the pros and cons of DNR. We felt that not having a DNR for this woman was cruel, and the family was not thinking about the woman's quality of life, but of themselves. Yes, it was hard to let someone die, but we need to examine our priorities.

Recently, my mother also died, and she refused to leave the house, call a doctor, or go to the hospital. Those were her wishes. Consequently, she suffered much more than if she had been treated palliatively at the hospital. It was very hard to accept her wishes. It was her body and she was competent mentally, so it was her decision. With no experience of nursing, the family found it was very hard to care for her. It was very difficult for all of us because what we wanted was her comfort. This time, the decision was selfishly dumping a burden on the helpless family who struggled to follow her wishes and perform the care she needed.

AFTER COMING HOME: JULY 2018

Amber was still experiencing a lot of pain when she came home from the hospital, but because it was the July long weekend, doctors were not available. The prednisone alone was not adequate for the pain. Doug and I took turns massaging Amber's back. It was so hot, and she seemed to be burning up, so we rubbed her back through her nightgown so the fabric would slide with our hands. She was experiencing so much pain that we called our friend Lisa, a physiotherapist, who agreed to see her. Lisa discovered that Amber was black and blue all down her back from our massages—a side effect of the prednisone. Lisa took a photo of her back and sent it to the family doctor, who discontinued the prednisone. I felt so badly that we had bruised her. Now Amber had *no* treatment at all.

Amber had to visit the chest clinic here in Barrie to discuss the Sarcoidosis and arrange a lung biopsy. It was getting harder for Amber to breathe and more exhausting for her to overcome the pain of dressing and going into the office. Amber probably didn't think she could have oxygen at home and didn't ask about it. I wondered why the physician hadn't thought of it. I was surprised by the delay of the biopsy. It would be mid-July before it was performed. I guess I watched too many medical shows on TV where biopsies were hurried along. In hindsight, I should have asked Amber to ask about the oxygen. I was not thinking of the possibilities of treatment at home with oxygen. I guess I was overwhelmed by her symptoms and the futility of visiting the hospital emergency.

During this time at home, we were still waiting for the gynecological consult that had originated in May. Most of Amber's pain was in the lower back near the pelvis. She lost her appetite even though I made her favourites, only to carry them back downstairs untouched. She stayed in her bedroom most of the time, getting sicker as the days progressed. We even went and got her pho because she wanted it, but she could only manage a few spoons of the soup. Amber was also vomiting. Doug and I would helplessly hear the retching, look at ourselves, and then go and clean up.

We learned that there was a shortage of gynecologists in Barrie at that time. We had to wait for our gynecologist to move to Barrie from the Maritimes. I liked the new gynecologist, but she couldn't get a biopsy within the office because Amber couldn't handle the pain. She also didn't have hospital privileges yet, so she couldn't do a biopsy with anesthetic in the hospital either, and the results would take a couple of weeks anyway. At least she gave Amber one of the most potent pain relievers you could get. I was disappointed. After waiting for a doctor, we get one with *no* hospital privileges! She couldn't admit Amber if needed. On our way to Southlake for the biopsy check-up the next week, the gynecologist phoned Amber to see how she was doing. At least she was concerned about the state of her health.

In mid-July, Amber was very weak the day we went to Southlake Hospital for the pre-op tests, and the drive tired her out. Many people thought we should have taken Amber to Toronto to visit an ED there in May. I knew the ED wait times were as long or longer down there, and we might not get any more satisfaction there. In retrospect, perhaps we should have gone to Toronto. I had yet to learn about the gynecologist shortage. Later, I learned that Barrie was the Regional Hospital for Women's Cancers. How could they be if they had no gynecologists?

Earlier this year in 2024, more than five years later, there were no gynecologists to cover emergencies for a day on a particular weekend. People were told to phone ER, and they would be told to go to Orillia or Newmarket. I guess gynecologists are still hard to find.

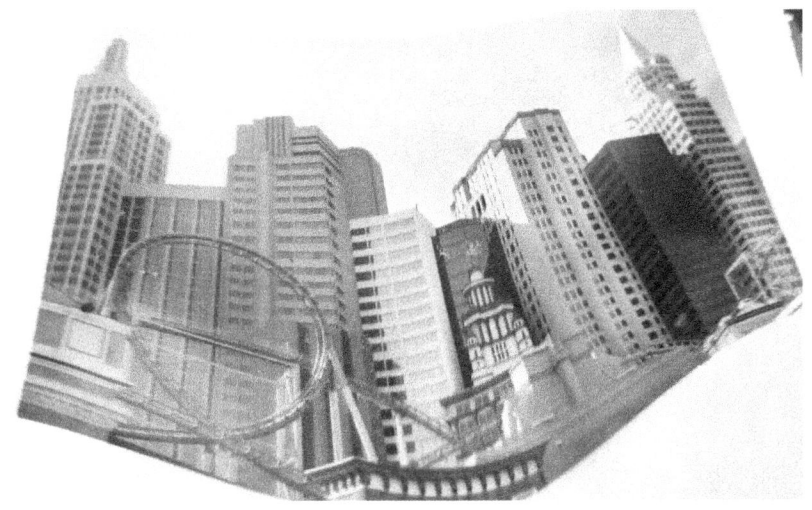

Amber's photo manipulation of her Las Vegas New York New York photo.

We felt like we were on a rollercoaster.

SOUTHLAKE

"To study philosophy is to learn to die." —Michel de Montaigne

The morning in mid-July when we arrived for the pre-biopsy work-up at Southlake Hospital in Newmarket, someone collapsed in the doorway to the clinic, blocking our access. We watched as the staff performed CPR and then, after he was revived, lift him to a bed. Amber was in a wheelchair all this time and was getting weaker by the second. We told the receptionist about Amber, and before they sent her down to the ED, they did vitals and took blood. She was chauffeured down to the ED and put directly into a bed! We had never been given a bed so quickly! Just as quickly, she was put on oxygen and given an IV and pain medication. She fell asleep almost instantly, and I was so thankful. I don't think she had slept for days. I was so grateful later in the afternoon when the ED aisles were full of waiting police and ambulance drivers standing by their patients, waiting to hand them off to the ER staff. So many people were waiting, which didn't include the walking wounded, who I couldn't see from where I was. I felt blessed.

We had arrived in Newmarket early in the morning, and I spent the afternoon glued to the monitors as if they were a television, watching the oxygen levels, heartbeat, blood pressure, and echocardiogram. At the same time, Amber mostly slept, waking only when she needed more pain medication. We didn't have a book because it was supposed to be a short visit. By supper, I had a migraine. I found a mini pharmacy in a device about the size of a vending machine. I video-conferenced with the pharmacist, who released dimenhydrinate and acetaminophen. I found a little canteen with sandwiches for Doug and me.

Amber went for a CT scan of her lungs, and I followed the orderly and waited in the hallway to return to the ED. I wondered why they were re-doing it. Later in the evening, Amber was moved into a small, quieter section of the ED, and it was implied that she would get admitted when a bed was available. She would stay here overnight and most of the next day. We finally saw a middle-aged female doctor close to midnight the first night, and I was grateful because we had had better experiences with the more mature doctors. The physician opened the dialogue with profuse apologies to both Amber and us. I guessed this didn't bode well. I wondered why the apologies when we could see how busy the ED was. It was then that we learned that the CT scan done in Barrie had been blurry, and that was why it was re-done. No, Amber did not have Sarcoidosis. (Dr. House and Amber's friends were right again.) I think the respirologist in Barrie was excited to get a relatively rare diagnosis and was too attached to that decision. The respirologist, a man, had not listened to my questions and requests. I asked about the pelvic pain and bleeding, and he ignored it as if it wasn't happening. He did state that "no—Sarcoidosis did not affect the uterus." If Doug had asked him those same questions, I had the feeling that he might have at least considered them. I felt that as a female patient, not all of Amber's symptoms were addressed, and as the female caregiver, I was not listened to. The new ED doctor in Southlake didn't tell us what the problem could be, or perhaps we were just too tired to hear it. I think they still weren't sure exactly what it was. We were told more tests would be done and Amber would be hospitalized. Knowing Amber would sleep comfortably that night, Doug and I left for the almost hour-long drive home.

The next day, we arrived in the morning because I did not want to miss the doctor. There had not been a visit so it didn't matter. Amber was sleeping, and we read the newspaper and books we had brought along. The oncologist came to speak with us. My worst fears seemed to be taking place. *An oncologist? Had I missed something?* I asked myself. Perhaps that was why we had so many apologies the night before. The oncologist only conferred with Doug and I because Amber was sleeping. Cancer was being investigated as a potential diagnosis. Both Doug and I were in shock, even though I had suspected cancer for some time. I had hoped that I was wrong.

Dr.Fung described cancer as this: "Cancer is, improbably, a disease unlike any other we've ever faced. It is not an infection. It is not an autoimmune disease. It is not a vascular disease. It is not a disease of toxins. Cancer is originally derived from our own cells but develops into an alien species," (2023).

Shortly after seeing the oncologist, Amber was transferred to a four-bed ward on the Oncology/Palliative Care Floor. It happened again on a Friday night, so only a few tests would be done on the weekend. I found it strange that there were both men and women in that room, but shrugged and thought it was what it was, and at least Amber had a bed.

Maté described personalities that were prone to various types of illnesses. He found that the patient who most commonly presented with malignancy was cooperative, appeasing, unassertive, did not express negative emotions, was excessively nice, pleasant to a fault, and were uncomplaining people pleasers." Amber was not all of these, but most of them. Amber was not entirely uncomplaining; she was assertive on subjects she was well versed in. Maté said they found cancer in the "stereotypical good girl." One who was "an over-achiever, top of the class, always pushing to develop talent or to be accepted by others," (2022). That was Amber. This is hard to take in—that our personalities can be so predictive of illnesses. Yet, they have studied and found this, and Amber fit the description.

Amber's oxygen tube was so long that she could get up and go to the bathroom alone. In only a few days, that changed. First, she fell and then had to be accompanied, and then she was catheterized. She had a catheter bag and no longer left the bed. It seemed as though the carcinoma moved onto a different place every day. It moved to her kidney, through her abdomen, and there were more tumours in her brain. Amber still did not have an official diagnosis, and I felt I was lying to her when I reassured her that we had to wait for the diagnosis. To this day, I am not sure that I did the right thing. They were investigating cancer, but they hadn't said for certain that was the diagnosis. I don't think cancer was in her thoughts. Her calcium became high, and the nurses restricted her water intake. Her metabolism was so high that she was projecting a lot of heat. There was also a fan going to cool her body down. Every day, my certainty that it was cancer increased.

A palliative care doctor monitored Amber's pain, and he told me that as Amber's breathing worsened, they would use a BIPAP to help. A BIPAP is a support system that provides a strong flow of air each time a patient inhales and does much of the work of breathing. It helps with mechanics, but it is still hard work. It is noisy, forceful, and blows one's lips apart. The palliative care doctor had a soft voice, and usually, I was standing to his right, which meant my deaf ear was closest. I didn't always hear the entire thing. When he told me about the BIPAP, the machine noise made it challenging to hear soft-spoken people. The room could get noisy with four people in beds and each with company.

The floor we were on had a rooftop patio and you could see the city of Toronto in the distance. One day, we tried to bring Amber, in a wheelchair, outside for the view and the nice weather. She only stayed a few minutes. The slight breeze was robbing her of breath even with the BIPAP.

I heard that Amber's lung X-ray was like popcorn. I wasn't exactly sure what that meant. Did it mean that all the air pockets in the lungs became filled with carcinoma, so there was no place for the air? Did the carcinoma fill her up with a solid mass? I wish I had seen the X-ray. I wanted to ask but was too intimidated to do so. Maybe it would make more sense to me. I so longed to read her chart. When I worked in the hospital, I could read my patient's charts when I had a question. I felt at a loss with the chart denied to me. Perhaps it would make it real. I still regret not asking.

Patients changed during the time in that ward, and one elderly lady was admitted. She must have had a serious infection because her sons were gowned and masked, or at least the mask was hanging around their necks as they strode back and forth, speaking on their phones. I thought this was odd. When my mother was in the hospital and contracted C. difficile, she was in an isolation room, and we had to wear gowns before going into the inner chamber and take the gowns off before we left the room so that we were not carrying the infection throughout the hospital. I had wondered why every patient was given a strong antibiotic which had been restricted in the hospital I had worked in, automatically on admission to that floor. Then, one evening, I found a map of the ward across from the nurse's station, and it showed which room had C. difficile, VRE, and other resistant bacterial infections. Maybe they didn't have enough isolation rooms in the hospital. It doesn't address the risk of the visitors in the room when people aren't following protocol. That elderly lady was one such patient. She would not stay in her bed and wandered through our curtains, wanting to converse even while her bare backside could be seen through her gown. We called nursing, and they put an alarm mat on the floor to notify them when she stepped out of bed. One afternoon, she took hold of Doug's head through the curtain and moved her hands up and down, trying to figure out what it was. It was funny, but that is how crowded it was.

Black humour started to be something that we used to diffuse the tension. One day, there was a *CODE RED* in the X-ray department, and all the connecting doors in the hallways were shut and locked. Doug said, in an unbelievable manner, that perhaps they had forgotten a patient on the X-ray bed and fried him by mistake. Unlikely as that was, Doug does tend toward the macabre. Typical Dad joke. Even fantasy entered Doug's dreams during this time. He had bizarre nightmares.

Finally, the team came in and told Amber that she had cancer—carcinoma, to be precise. Carcinoma is a solid cancer; a tumour. Amber started crying, and I quickly went to one side and grabbed her hand, and the palliative care doctor took the other. Later, she told her father that she was sad that she wouldn't be able to have children. She did not have an idea about the seriousness of her condition. She didn't know the prognosis and neither did we. We, again, felt helpless because we didn't have clear answers and did not want to scare her if we were wrong, so we didn't tell her that death was imminent. They did not know the type of carcinoma or where the primary was, so they couldn't give us any more details. Doug became frustrated with the team because they wouldn't explain the prognosis. Kalanithi said, "The reason doctors don't give patients specific prognoses was not merely because they cannot . . . Getting into statistics is like trying to quench thirst with salty water. The angst of facing mortality has no remedy in probability," (2016).

When the carcinoma reached her neck region, they could do a biopsy without causing too much strain on Amber. I think they said it was endometrial carcinoma, or maybe it was multiple myeloma. The team rushed in and tried to find a mole or spot on Amber's skin, so I am unsure. When I asked the family doctor many months afterward, he said it was pelvic carcinoma. We were never really told clearly what this thing was, that was killing our daughter. Near the end of July, Amber was informed that nothing could be done for her. At this time, a DNR was suggested, and we all quickly said yes, we wanted that. I think it surprised the team. I bet they often have to explain what would happen without one. I guess that experience within the Barrie hospital occurred to encourage a long conversation about it. The doctors told us if Amber's friends wanted to see her, they needed to hurry up and come quickly. I asked the doctors to stop the antibiotics when we had decided Amber was palliative. She didn't need the side effects of them. Amber was moved onto the palliative side and had her own room soon after that. From then on, I stayed at the hospital, sleeping on a fold-away bed, which became a chair during the day.

Amber and I went through her phone directory, and I had heard of many of her friends. Amber bravely and calmly phoned and told most of them that she was dying. I was awed by the strength it took. Sometimes, she would tell them she would see them in a month or two, and I would have to take the phone into the hallway and explain that there were only days left. The carcinomas in her brain were affecting her memory. I listened to her friends explain how Amber had changed their lives by giving them confidence, a resume, editing their thesis, or something of that nature. I wondered if Amber was so smart and helpful and changed lives for the better, why hadn't she been able to find another job in the art world? Why couldn't she get a full-time job, period? This was bittersweet, I was soothing their tears on the phones while my own heart was breaking. I felt like I should be the one crying, but crying only happened months after I finished executing her will. I disassociated so that I would get things done. David Kessler, a grief therapist, said that shock gives the griever time to adjust to what follows, and I think I was in shock for a long time (2019).

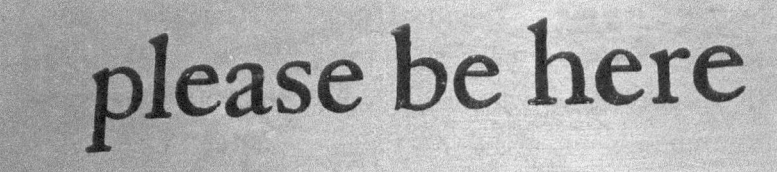

One of Amber's signs for her sign project.

Prior to that moment when the doctors said to get the friends there quickly, I had wondered where Amber's friends were. Why weren't the friends visiting her in the hospital? I had even wondered why they hadn't seen her at home. I discovered that friends had wanted to come, but that Amber had nixed the idea. I was glad that I had figured out her phone because Amber had more growths on her brain, and she couldn't always do it.

Come, her friends did. It seemed like they came out of the woodwork. One came from Vancouver. One took the subway, the GO train, and trekked to the hospital (the hospital was not close). That friend came with roti, which had always been the menu choice when they went to celebrate Amber's birthday. She only found a big tablespoon in the kitchen, and Amber called her a goddess. Amber dug right in and ate a mouthful, but that was all that she could eat. Maybe someone else could have eaten some if Amber had not taken from the middle. Amber ate very little now. Even yogurt and ice cream were both forsaken by her. The lady who brought the meal trays tried to entice Amber with something to eat. Amber said she wanted cake one day, and the lady found some. Amber put her finger into the icing and savoured it but didn't eat any more of it. I was so thankful to this woman. She tried to make Amber's last days comfortable in her own way.

One of Amber's last requests was for whipped cream, which I asked my sister if she could bring some—it could just be a can of whipped cream—as Amber wasn't eating. My sister brought fancy Italian pastries, and Amber poked her finger into the whipped cream and tasted it but did not eat the pastry. We searched for Sweet Tarts when Sweet Tarts was the wish.

That same friend who had brought the roti returned with a Himalayan salt lamp and a very long creeping plant. She placed the plant into the window and draped it so that Amber could reach out and touch it. She hauled all that on the subway/GO and on foot. Other friends came with beautiful flowers, handmade cards made by their children, and some candy. One friend brought a handmade rosary, which she had made from amber beads, crying as she threaded them. There were also stuffed animals and a crocheted animal. One friend brought a spray of cedar with lavender and a ribbon. One friend came in and ran out crying. The people from work came and cried the whole time. I saw that everyone loved Amber, and they were very nice and thoughtful. There were more memories for me to cherish. How her life was important, and she was more successful than she realized. It is hard to watch someone die and harder if that person felt their life had not been successful. Their lives were cut short and there is no opportunity to turn life around. But that wasn't Amber's reality from my perspective. This last statement was very important to me. As Amber's health declined and her future was removed, thoughts of failure were uppermost in her mind. I didn't really see failure though. I saw a life that had touched many lives; that she had helped many, and there was a large group of friends who really cared for her. She met Whitman's new view of success.

I finally understood what it meant in the Christmas story when Mary listened to the Wise Men and held their words in her heart. I was doing what Mary had done and I am still holding all the love they expressed. It made her death a little easier to accept.

Doug phoned one of our friends whose wife was a lawyer and asked if she could prepare a will for Amber and get her signature as soon as possible while she was still competent. The lawyer came and tested Amber for competency, and Amber signed the will. If it had been the next day, Amber might not have passed the test. That was how quickly everything was changing. For some reason, I was made the executor of the will.

Until the doctors had urged her friends to come, Amber hadn't let work know how sick she was. They said they needed a new doctor's note the week before. We told the nurses that Amber was still eligible for sick benefits from the government, and we had no idea what debts were outstanding, so we needed to ensure sick benefits were forthcoming. The hospital social worker wrote the sick note, and I angrily delivered it. When asked how she was, I answered *"worse than you know"* and left abruptly.

Amber and I planned her funeral, what music she wanted, and other arrangements. We decided (mostly me—to cut down on postage) that it should be a celebration of life, and the gifts would be *from* her. We tried to remember her belongings, which were brand new, still in the original packaging, because Amber had been saving for an apartment. All the future plans that were made, like returning to school in September and a new apartment, would now go unrealized. All that planning and waiting for her life to improve, only to lose it before she could make it happen. We made a list of names, and most close friends and relatives got something. My mother and sister came in while we were working on this, and my mother was appalled. She thought Amber should not have to go through this but left unspoken that Amber should not be dying before her grandmother and her mother. My family was the type to squash down feelings and ignore reality. Perhaps I shouldn't have had the idea of wrapping it all. Wrapping was time-consuming, especially as we made remembrance cards and wrote thank-you notes.

Before Amber was made palliative, and was still in the four-bed ward, she would call at five a.m. and ask us to come, and I always put her off. As I have said before, I have Fibromyalgia with chronic pain, and I was afraid that if I didn't get some rest, I would crash and be useless. I didn't realize how drastically she changed with each passing night and the terrors she was experiencing during the night. In hindsight, maybe I should have stayed over sooner, but the room was so overcrowded, and I needed to pace myself.

Amber was seeing and hearing things. Was it the high dose of narcotics needed to relieve her pain or the tumours in her brain? Or could it have been the dying process? When I did stay, I spent most nights with her hand gripping mine. Many of the hallucinations were of saving the world. One time, she and her sister Molly needed to sing a verse of a song they didn't entirely remember, or the world was going to end. I thought of her art and the project as a superhero. She was still trying to save the world as she was dying. I thought it showed Amber's goal to help people. Another time, I walked in after getting coffee, and Amber told me that the choir director was angry because we didn't have the songs perfect. Amber loved music and had piano, guitar, composing, and vocal lessons. As a child, she sang herself to sleep. I had to remove one stuffed animal from the hospital bed because it was bad-mouthing her and asking her to do evil things. Other times, the *"bad"* people were outside the hospital window telling her to do bad things, and she didn't want to. Images like Amber was experiencing, or dark images like the Grim Reaper, are among the images that can appear (Moody and Perry, 2023).

Delirium is common at the end of life and could be a sign of dehydration as well as the painkillers. Apparently, it is odd for a patient to remain mentally clear during the final stages of malignant illness (quoted in Moody and Perry, 2023).

Repetition of speech is very common during the delirium and Smartt found they often expressed themes such as gratitude and resistance to death (2017). The language used by those near to death is very often metaphorical and the dying person may have trouble understanding figurative language. Anthropologists do not find the language of metaphor everywhere. To receive famous last words during a moment of lucidity just before dying is a romantic notion (Erard, 2019). Emotion is also increased with repetition. The second repeat exposes the meaning, and the third time, it gives tone and pitch and connects to a non-verbal world. Drama and intensive emotion are created with repetition (Smartt, 2017).

I also thought of the Bible passage of the gold undergoing heat to strengthen it, and that had comforted me when my dad died. I thought these visions were testing Amber. Another time, Amber said a group of people were circling her bed, and there was a man with a funny face but you shouldn't leave him with young children.

There are many anecdotes of pre-deceased ancestors or friends circling the bed when someone is dying. It is felt they have appeared to help their relative through the death process. When my mother died recently, she saw her mother by the bedside. Mom told my sister incredulously that her mother was still alive.

One question that did come up during the day was what would happen to *"her"* when she died. She meant her spirit or her consciousness. I quickly said that I thought God wanted her in heaven early to be an angel and help people from above, but that got rejected by Amber. Amber was no longer Catholic—she was now an atheist, I think. What do you tell an atheist about what happens after death? My daughters, raised in the faith, lapsed when a thoughtless priest said gays were not welcome in the church. My daughters had friends within the LBTQIA+ group. Who in their right mind says such a controversially negative thing at Christmas and Easter when people who aren't at mass throughout the year show up? Let alone the un-Christian spirit in that statement. Another time, a different priest said everyone was welcome in the church and we were supposed to be kind and treat everyone with respect. My daughters did not hear that priest though.

Apparently, asking *"what happens to me?"* is an age-old question going back to even Plato's day. It is one of the most commonly asked questions to clergy and hospice workers. The soul, by definition in *Encarta Dictionary*, is the whole of human attributes that manifest as consciousness, thought, feeling, and will. It thought to be distinct from the physical body and religious soul. Many systems of religion believe this consciousness continues to exist after death.

Sam Dresser in Aeon wrote an essay entitled "How Not to Fear Your Death." In it, he said the fear of death was "at an existential level, brought on by the almost unthinkable notion that there is, and only ever will be, one of you, a fleeting speck of an event in the infinite history of the Universe." Furthermore, he wrote that death was considered "the great deprivation." Death takes away the future and "its possibility of aging into wisdom and a 'full life,'" (2020). Amber had just been admitted into a paralegal course at Georgian College and should have started in September. The fees were already paid. She had been hoping that she would be able to get her life back on track and change her future from the dreary cashier job that Amber had performed during the past two years and for which she was highly overqualified. One of her friends thought she should go to law school instead, but I think she was afraid of the debt load. Amber was being robbed of her future.

Nabokov said, "Our existence is but a crack of light between two eternities of darkness." Amber had studied philosophy. She should have known this, or at least better than I, but in the dying process, do you really think of philosophy? Perhaps she did, and that darkness was overwhelming. People her age don't think they will die soon, and therefore, don't meditate on it. Death should not be feared, Dresser wrote, because it was neither uncomfortable nor painful to be dead. Death is an absence (2020). The act of dying is another matter. Dr. Kalanithi described these feelings as he was dying and debilitated: "My imagined future and my identity collapsed, and I faced the same existential quandaries my patients faced," (2016). Amber was not alone with this question: *where would she go?* A friend of hers discussed this question using the Stoics as an example. He studied philosophy too. He was better prepared than I for this question, I thought. We asked the Chaplain on the floor if there was another answer that might calm Amber's fears. She used Indigenous peoples' death mythology. I don't know whether it satisfied Amber or not. This fear of death and nightmarish nights showed me why my father feared being alone during the nights before his death when he was still at home. He kept my mother and brother up, but this happened long before he was put into palliative care. Amber had just learned about her imminent death while in the hospital, but Dad had many months to stew about it.

Many cultures have heaven, hell, underworld, pure-land and others, which provide a where and when for the living to consider. This question is so common globally that O'Connor, a neuroscientist, thought it might be "an indication that the strong desire to search for and map the whereabouts of our loved ones (the desire to have them here and now) is biologically based." She felt that "the biological evidence is embedded in the brain" and hypothesized perhaps within the hippocampus (2022).

In the song "THE WAY," the group, Fastball, tells a story of a couple. It is such a happy lilting song that I was surprised by the subject matter when I looked up the song. The song is actually about a couple who goes missing and died. I was totally deceived by the happy-sounding bridge, which actually was what Fastball thought death might be like, or what it might be in heaven. The roads would be all paved in gold, the people would never be cold because the sun always shined. They would never be hungry, and they'll never age anymore. No one knows what happens when we die because no one comes back to tell us. We can only conjecture.

One evening, I talked to my friend while Amber slept, and she strongly recommended the *Sacrament of the Sick* for Amber. Doug had previously broached this subject several times with Amber, and she had said *NO*. I told my friend this, but she held firm and wanted me to do it while Amber slept—or at least a second baptism. I said I would not go against Amber's wishes, and my friend's husband came on the phone and tried to convince me of the importance of this rite. They said it was *necessary* so that Amber would go to heaven. I felt that Amber had a good heart, and she had helped many people during her lifetime and should get into heaven on her own merit. It was a disturbing conversation. People don't need a second baptism. I thought if I had gone against Amber's wishes, the sacrament wouldn't work because she didn't want it. Thank goodness only one friend mentioned this.

Why do some people get to have their life prolonged and complete their bucket list or sell their belongings so their funeral gets paid? Why did Amber die so quickly? Some people like my father would not get the cancer identified, and perhaps, had he, he might have lived a little longer. He had just said no to any intervention, but death came slowly. He lived almost five months longer.

One night, when Amber needed something, I left the room and was surprised that in the quiet, dark hallway there was a very long line of people. *Very* long and very quiet. They were there to say goodbye to a patriarch, uncle, brother, or whatever the relationship was. It was eerily quiet. You could feel the people's respect for the process and for all those sleeping in the hospital.

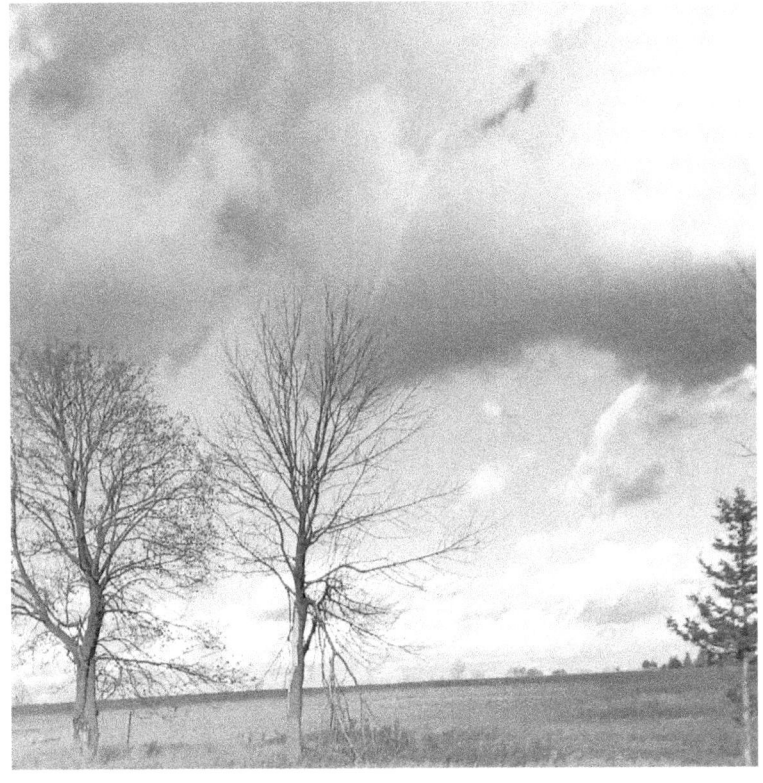

Storm clouds ahead.

DEATH

"Some deaths are traumatic when accompanied by exposure to the loved one's physical agony, medical procedures, and suddenness."

—David Kessler

In less than a week after getting the diagnosis, Amber complained of leg pain, and her legs moved restlessly over the bed. The nurses were busy, so I texted my friend, the physiotherapist, who suggested heat. You can't get a hospital heating pad, but they have warmed blankets. I went to and fro—getting warm blankets from the warming oven. Then Amber pulled her oxygen mask off, and I called the nurse because I couldn't get her to keep it on. The nurse told me it was terminal agitation, "It happens just before you die," she said. Now, I had a choice. Let her suffer through the restless legs and not being able to breathe, or sedate her such that she was comfortable but probably in a coma. Doug had gone home, so I called him—"What should I tell the nurse? Could you please come to the hospital?" I opted for sedation. It was my goal to keep Amber as comfortable as possible. Doug arrived and stayed that night, and no hallucinations bothered Amber. Amber lay there peacefully, looking like she was sleeping. It reminded me of when she was an infant. She just looked like she was not sick.

Now that she was in a coma, she still had two more visitors. One was a friend who had done a *Nuit Blanche* project with her and whose father was in the same hospital, also dying of cancer. Amber and she had just figured out the day before that it was the same hospital. While she was there, I made sure I was always touching Amber. Otherwise, during the day, I read to her, talked, and tried to keep a connection. Amber's old boyfriend and another woman were the last to visit Amber. I didn't know he was coming, or I would have told him ahead of time in case he wanted to save the trip from Guelph. As he visited, I kept my hands on Amber's feet. I tried to reassure her that I was still there.

As I wrote earlier, one of Amber's friends had brought a spray of cedar and lavender tied in a bow. There was another flower, too, but I forget which one. When I got up the following day, I smudged Amber with it, but it was not lit. Then I sat down and started reading to her. Nurses came in shortly afterwards to prepare for shift change, and I walked up to see about changing books. One of the nurses came into that room and said I needed to come right back, and we ran back to the room, and Amber was pronounced dead. I said, "if you didn't like the book, you just had to say so"—bad humor at the wrong time. Just then, my sister texted me to see if Amber was okay. I called her and asked, "how did you know?" It was the *exact* time! Then I called Doug and told him. Amber died August 1, 2018. The journey was four months long.

Now, it was time to wait. I told Amber not to worry about us, we would be okay, but to move along to the white light to something better. I placed the cedar spray into her hands. I wasn't sure how okay we would be, but I wanted Amber to stop suffering. After seven a.m., I called Amber's friend in Burlington and gave her the bad news and the same news to another friend in Toronto. The Toronto friend called back and asked if they could put the information on Facebook now. While she was alive, Amber didn't want it on Facebook, but the social media saved me so many phone calls. So many people replied to the Facebook revelation, and they said wonderful things.

My sister and her partner arrived before Doug could make it to the hospital, and we packed up flowers and gifts, my belongings, and said goodbye to Amber. I led the procession up the hall, but halfway up, I wanted to turn back. We couldn't leave without her! I could see the orderly with the bed for the morgue slip down the other hallway, trying to hide the stretcher from us. When I saw that, I knew I couldn't take up more time from staff. We said our goodbyes and thanks at the Nursing Station, then left.

I believe it was the breathlessness that caused Amber's death. They had adjusted her oxygen to the highest it would go. Yet, the carcinoma in her lungs was probably not the primary site. Kalathini said that only 0.0012% of thirty-six-year-olds get lung cancer. So Amber was in a very small percentage since she was only thirty-four (2016). Afterwards, while organizing Amber's things, I found a handmade button that read *Boycott Breathing*. That button made me stop and think. Why would Amber make a stupid button like that? Was it just a coincidence that I found it then? Why would she think it was funny?

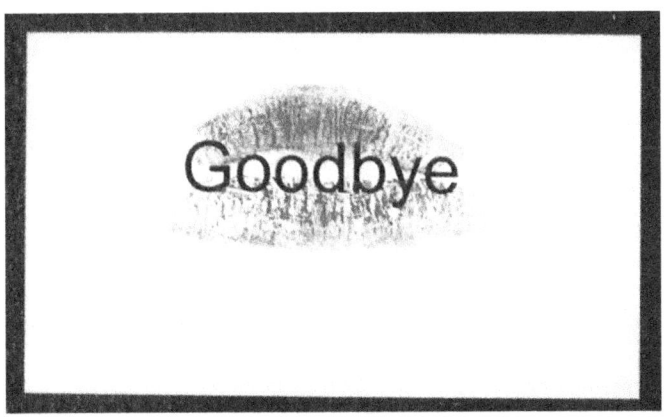

One of Amber's Break-Up Kisses project

OBESITY AND CANCER

Half of the adult population is overweight. For the majority, severe obesity is incurable without drugs or surgery. Obesity is often mistaken as a disease of excessive calories, but in fact, it has been found to be a mainly hormonal disorder of too much insulin (Fung, 2020). Fung, an endocrinologist in Toronto, said that the generation born in 1980s and 1990s are the heaviest generation, but their risks of cancer exceed those people of comparable weights in different generations.

Chris van Tullekin, in *Ultra Processed People: Why We Can't Stop Eating Food That Isn't Food,* felt that some of the obesity we are finding globally "comes from the collision of some ancient genes with a new food ecosystem that is engineered to drive excess consumption, and that we currently seem to be unable, or perhaps, unwilling to improve," (2023). Even though obesity was thought as a disease of excess, it seems malnutrition is often present. Genetic vulnerability, poverty, injustice, inequality, trauma, fatigue, and stress are also related to the rise of obesity. Many of the above situations show deeper societal problems which put a person at risk of obesity. If we decreased poverty, we could prevent a lot of lung cancer and obesity, Van Tulleken thought. Maté felt that obesity was a marker of internal stress and that most neo-liberal countries had more obesity and therefore, he felt that obesity was a marker for an international stress epidemic (2022).

Obesity is stigmatizing and many people end up living with obesity as their identity instead of living with a disease. Although forty-two percent of Americans are affected with obesity, Dorothea Vafidis wrote, in *How Bias and Stigma Affects Patients*, that it was still socially acceptable to have bias against those with obesity. A large part of the population is "vulnerable to blatant and unfair treatment, and this bias is perpetuated in the media," (2022). Fat-shaming can actually cause the patient to gain more weight from the stress.

I knew society had a bias against women and the obese, but I guess I held the physician up to a higher standard. Within the medical community, bias against obesity is more ingrained than any other bias, and is a huge barrier to care. In fact, some primary care providers view people with obesity as non-compliant and therefore, spend less time with them and provide less kind, supportive, or compassionate care. Dusenbury said women reported that any time they visited the doctor, all their complaints were blamed on their weight (2018). I felt that Amber was being blamed for her weight and could see what I thought was disgust on some of the younger male doctors' faces, but I told myself that I was imagining it. Fung felt that we actually should be looking more closely to people with obesity because of the cancer risks that were found after 2005. Cancers such as liver, endometrial, esophageal, kidney, colorectal, pancreatic, multiple myeloma, and breast cancer all increased in people with obesity. This points out that stigmatizing patients with obesity may be increasing their risks of cancer (2022).

Those people born in 1985 have five times the risk of kidney cancer. Compared with a non-smoker, a BMI over forty has an eighty-eight percent increase for cancer. BMI's have been found to be a crude measure and it has been found that fifty-seven percent of women who were labelled overweight were metabolically healthy. All of the cancers that a person with obesity is at risk for, make up forty percent of all cancers.

It wasn't the 2000s that the risk of cancer with obesity was recognized. In his book, *The Cancer Code: A Revolutionary Understanding of a Medical Mystery*, Fung delves into the idea that cancer can be linked with insulin. The National Health and Nutrition Examination Survey database of 1999 suggested high insulin levels more than doubles the risk of cancer, regardless of the weight. Non-diabetic, non-obese people with high insulin had a *two hundred and fifty percent* increased risk of cancer deaths. People with Type 2 Diabetes, with insulin as treatment, have a *forty-four percent* increased risk of cancer than those treated with Metformin because the Metformin does not increase levels of insulin. Sulfonylureas used to be the first choice of therapy, but are now linked to a *thirty-six percent* increase in cancer.

Insulin is a highly potent growth factor, and it has been found that tall people have higher incidences of cancer because, it is thought, of the higher levels of growth factors. It has been found that cancer cells have more insulin cell receptors on the cell membrane. This can affect the growth and metabolism of the cancer cells.

Despite intensive investigations, in five percent of cancer cases, the primary site cannot be determined, even on autopsy. Metastases happens earlier than previously thought. In fact, we could have cells that have undergone mutations when we are healthy but the healthy killer cells in our body usually stop them from growing.

Fatty liver causes chronic inflammation and as was discussed earlier, inflammation can affect the immune system which would normally kill these rogue cancer cells. Inflammation from chronic stress can damage DNA and its repair. It may also activate genes that support the growth and support tumour cells. Inflammation can stimulate blood vessels to increase so they can bring nutrients to the tumour cells (Maté, 2022). Inflammation can also affect the body's ability to fight pathogens. The inflammation can lead to cirrhosis and cancer. Over the past forty years, liver cancer has tripled, and death has more than doubled. Pancreatic cancer has increased one percent every year from 2006 to 2016. If people feel threatened or insecure, especially over an extended period of time, our bodies are programmed to turn on inflammation, Maté claimed. Although the USA "celebrates itself as the wealthiest in history, Wade Davis, an anthropologist, wrote in Rolling Stone magazine that most Americans live on a high wire, with no safety net to brace a fall," and "middle-class families are working longer, managing all kinds of stress, and shouldering greater financial risk than previous generations," (Maté, 2022). The current times, with wars and inflation, after the COVID epidemic, and insecurity in governments, are certainly putting a lot of people under a lot of stress and that may be reflected in the incidence of cancer in young people rising.

Cancer found in Duchess Kate Middleton has led to articles about cancer in young people. The rates have shot up seventy-nine percent in people from 204 countries, and death from cancer has increased to twenty-eight percent in a 2023 study reported in the *BMJ Oncology*. The cause is unknown, but factors that may contribute to the increase may be obesity, environmental factors producing toxic chemicals in the food and water, as well as poor sleep, alcohol, and tobacco use. Early screening that includes genetic testing may play a part, and many organizations are calling for screening guidelines to have lower age requirements. Our processed food and overuse of antibiotics could also have changed the viruses and bacteria that make up our GUT microbiome. Processed food and antibiotics have been linked to inflammation, which in turn can lead to cancer. Cancer is, improbably, a disease unlike any other we have ever faced, Fung felt. "It is not an autoimmune disease. It is not a vascular disease. It is not a disease of toxins. Cancer is originally derived from our own cells but develops into an alien species," (2022).

AFTERMATH

"When a person is born, we rejoice, and when they're married, we jubilate, but when they die, we try to pretend nothing happened."

—Margaret Mead

In *The Year of Magical Thinking*, Joan Didion was afraid that after her husband's return from the dead, he would need his shoes (2005). We didn't take long to clean Amber's closets and bookshelves. We had to find the items that Amber had delineated be given to specific friends before the Celebration of Life. We didn't know what debts Amber left us. We had the storage locker rent as an added expense and needed to make room for the belongings stored there. We did this with deep, dark circles under our eyes, looking and acting like we were in shock.

I was so afraid that I would cry at the Celebration of Life. Amber's former place of work, *XPACE*, rented a bus for the people from Toronto so they could come to the Celebration of Life. There was a large crowd of people. Some of her university friends from Guelph all arranged to wear a hat to honour Amber's obsession with hats. Near the end of the evening, I stood alone in the middle of the hall, forlornly watching a child play with one of Amber's friends. I was lost and sad that no grandchildren would be in my life.

After death, society reinforces denial, Heath said, which can gently cushion the mind for some time (2015). We are not that powerful to stay in denial, and nor should we avoid grieving. We have to face grieving at some time. Being denied the chance to grieve can result in anger, which we are conditioned to believe we have no right to experience. Fromm said, "Grief is the experience and natural feelings that come from loss." We have trouble not experiencing grief. If one "wanted to be spared from grief at all costs," it would require that person not to have experienced love, and this totals detachment; "It would exclude the ability to experience happiness," (quoted in Kessler, 2019).

I needed her belongings to mean something to someone, or to help others. Cleaning out took longer than necessary because I wanted good homes for the items. We brought most of the clothes to Value Village, but the big heavy winter coat she had just bought was brought to the homeless shelter. We were kept busy ferrying belongings from one mission store to another. We found out that the library would take a box of books a week, but after a few drop-offs, they informed us they wanted only fiction from then on. I had brought non-fiction art books and philosophy books to them in prior weeks. We brought books to the used bookstore, but they required an appointment and limited the number of boxes you could bring. (Yes, there were that many boxes—Amber was a reader.) Her excuse for not using the library in Toronto, when I had confronted her years before when she lived in Toronto, was a fear of bedbugs. I learned afterwards that the library had procedures to rid books of bedbugs. They used dogs who could smell the bugs. Some books went to the missions, some to the church rummage sale (cookbooks), and some cookbooks were donated to the local cooking program at the high school. I tried to give some books to Georgian College, but they have a limited library and required an itemized list ahead of time, which took too long. Georgian College has mostly a digital library. We even tried the OCADU, from which Amber had graduated with her Master of Fine Art, but they weren't interested either. Some books had never been opened. I put the cooking magazines on a table on the lawn by the sidewalk for people to help themselves. We were kept busy for four months going through belongings and giving them away. I even found all of Amber's favourite stuffed toys from childhood and kept the baby Care Bear.

My mother's belongings, after she died recently, were not treated to these long, tedious trips. For one, there was no one home to answer any phone calls and dispense with the objects. They had a finite time to pack up. I convinced them not to throw out the wheelchair. I wanted it to be donated. I found it hard to watch things just being dumped into a dump bin, but at the same time, they were *just* things. Things that my mother had saved for years, thrown into a bin because no one wanted the McDonald's toy collection, a collection Mom had spent years collecting and talking about. These toys were still in their wrappers. My nephew, as a child, played with them in the wrappers. Mostly looking at all of them. No one had the time or energy to try and sell them on E-Bay, or room to store them until they could sell them. Yet, I felt it wasn't environmentally responsible.

Losing Amber had changed my priorities. Who cares if your driveway is a little scraped by the snowplough when you have lost a child? Yet, my finding good homes for her belongings was a little hypocritical. The realization that things were not as important came after I had given the items away and finished all my duties as an executor. That came when I truly started to grieve.

Banking was another matter. Amber's banks were all online, and those banks could not make estate accounts. The brick-and-mortar banks would only open estate accounts for people who had accounts in the branch. Even the online bank's parent company's brick-and-mortar bank, would not help us. Yet, all the government, insurance, and other cheques were made out to the estate of Amber Landgraff. How to cash the cheques became an issue. Our bank allowed it because we had enough funds to cover any bad cheques and with the request of the Financial Planner. All the banks required a death certificate and a copy of the will. The online bank had each part of her accounts in a different location, and they all needed copies of the will and death certificate. Even after receiving the required paperwork, they would keep the amounts of her debts and savings private from me, the executor. They would not tell me the exact amounts within her accounts. To deal with them required several months and many phone calls and faxes.

Her cellphone also required the will and death certificate. Even after I supplied the paperwork, they couldn't tell me whether we owed money or not. I finally went to the storefront, and the clerk behind the counter was on the phone with the head office for several hours before the account was closed and paid in full. Even Apple required the death certificate and will to open her computer, iPod, and phone so we could use them. They wanted a probated will, but the will was simple, and probate was unnecessary. Thank goodness the lawyer had put a clause in the will about the computers and equipment being inherited by us. People have died without this clause and have had to take Apple to court. I was annoyed. The equipment was purchased and belonged to someone, no longer by the manufacturer. If you didn't win the court case, the equipment was useless. We buy the equipment from a store, not rent it. They should not have had that much clout. I felt they were intrusive.

Even Facebook requires a beneficiary, or you are locked out of your loved one's account. So many of Amber's friends had put condolences on her social media page that the program recognized that she was dead before we could delete the account, and Facebook made it *In Memoriam*. We also cannot close my father's account even though he has nothing on his Facebook page, except for a little blue head when you look for his name. After learning that, we quickly made beneficiaries on our own social network accounts.

Then, there was the sick pay that was owed before Amber died. Amber had started the paperwork but had not filled it out each week because she was so ill. I went to the *Employment Services* office and told them my long, sad story and how the tumours on Amber's brain had made it impossible to finish the paperwork. I brought the will and death certificate and paperwork from her employer. The woman at the desk helped fill out the required paperwork and then said she would send it, and it would be assessed if Amber was sick enough to receive the money. "That she was *sick enough!*" I exclaimed. "*How much sicker could someone be if they died?*" I started to cry. In the end, she was assessed, and we received the back pay in the estate of Amber Landgraff.

When you die, your student loan is forgiven, but a copy of the death certificate and will is required for that also. That was very easily solved with a phone call and a fax.

By the end of December, we had emptied the storage locker and paid that bill. Time for the natural grieving happened in the New Year.

GRIEF

"A wife who loses a husband is called a widow. A husband who loses a wife is a widower. A child who loses his parents is an orphan. There is no word for a parent who loses a child. Lose your child and you're . . . nothing."

—*Tennessee William*

We should not be surprised if we see and feel the presence of a dead loved one, O'Connor said (2022). It can explain how our brain functions normally. There are maps within the brain with a code for each location to help us keep track of where we are in the world, but also where other important things and people are in the world. We are unaware of developing shortcuts in the brain for routines. The more the shortcut is used, the stronger and bigger the pathway. Sometimes, this becomes evident in reading and music. It has been shown that the letters don't have to be in proper order as long as the first and last letters are in the right place, the brain can read them accurately. In music, we sometimes anticipate the following note's sound. This anticipation also happens when we are moving around familiar landscapes. We arrive somewhere and are unsure how we got there because the brain directs us to go automatically. The brain "also maps where the loved one is and will search for them when they are gone," (O'Connor, 2022). When we come home, for example, the brain anticipates our loved one to be in their usual place, and this phenomenon explains why, after death, we see or feel their presence even though they have died. For the brain, your loved one is simultaneously gone, but also everlasting in the well-worn pathways in the brain's circuitry. You are walking through two worlds at the same time. Grief happens when there is a mismatch between what the brain expects and the reality, that the loved one can no longer be found in space or time. This premise makes no sense for the brain, which is confused and upset. It takes the brain longer to learn the pathways may still be there, but the person doesn't exist anymore. After not finding the loved one often enough, the loved one will no longer be predicted by the brain. It is comforting that the Amber still exists in the brain because she lived and was loved, and the pathway will continue to be there despite not being used. Although Amber is no longer in the physical world, she still exists in the wiring neurons of my brain. O'Connor hypothesized the memory might be in the hippocampus. Seeing our loved ones is a common phenomenon and doesn't mean we are going crazy. I admit also that I experienced these feelings and illusions. I thought Amber came and hugged me as I was going to bed. Often, before she was sick, Amber would come into the bedroom and sit with us, and we would play *Rocket Racoon* on the tablet. When I felt her presence, I was comforted and awed. It seemed magical and I was afraid to tell people of the experience. I also felt this after our dog died recently. I could feel her weight as if curled up at my feet. I am disappointed that these experiences were just electricity moving through my brain.

Grief was expected to be shocking to Didion, but she did not expect it to be "obliterative, dislocating to both mind and body. We might expect to be prostrate inconsolable and crazy with grief. We don't expect to be crazy, cool customers who believe their husband is about to return and need his shoes," (2005). I dreamt that Amber died but she returned alive the next day and returned home. I was surprised by this miracle, and she continued to live as she had previously. Amber was no longer sick. No, she did not become a zombie. Today, I can still remember how real it seemed. It was so vivid and full of details.

I still occasionally dream of Amber. Usually, the dreams are shopping trips or party planning. Events that are pleasant. Sometimes she is helping me in the dream.

Grief affects hormones, the immune system, the lymphatic system, and the hematological system, Maté said (2022). The risk of malignancy, skin, and lung cancer increases during grieving, and the chance for Multiple Sclerosis doubles. Yet, Heath said, "Grief is not a disease or disorder or pathology," (2015). The griever is pale with dark circles under the eyes, and experiences fatigue, eats more or eats less, has digestive disorders, depression, palpitations, tremors, hair loss, migraines, and sympathy pains. I had dark circles under my eyes when we were still in the hospital. I had never had such dark circles, and it looked like the bags under my eyes had bags under them. That winter, I cried and cried. I ate too much, thinking there was no reason not to. It was as though I was swallowing my unhappiness, eating my way through the pain. Life goes so quickly, why not enjoy it while you can? Why deny the gratification of chocolate? I didn't sew any of my projects any longer. I didn't do anything. My asthma was worse, and there have been physician visits over the past five years for palpitations, tremors, migraines, and digestive issues, just like Heath said. I read Heath recently, five years later. With loss, Heath wrote that we could experience a "decrease in self-esteem, lack of self-confidence, loss of future dreams, and loneliness." Our seeming loss of a future can cause anger and grief, and we also lose the bond with the past. I felt this loss of the future. Why celebrate Christmas anymore? There is no future. Why keep these books that Molly won't want? There is no future. O'Connor wrote, in *The Grieving Brain*, that when the world changes suddenly, like when a loved one dies, utter confusion can occur. "The confusion is not as simple as denial, although that may be how others describe it.

Instead, it's the utter disorientation people experience in acute grief," (2022). I lived like this for a long time. My grief became my constant companion and then evolved into complex grief. I gave away books that I regret now, and I think I tore up my Masters project. It has been said that no major decisions should be made for at least six months after a death because of this confusion. We signed a contract that we shouldn't have. I wondered why I was still alive. Didion wrote that she hadn't realized how different real grief was compared to how she had imagined it: "The unending absence that follows, the void, the very opposite of meaning, the relentless succession of moments during which we experience, we will confront the experience of meaninglessness itself," (2005). Bruce Perry said that the loss of meaningfulness was "excruciatingly painful." Grief was also said to be a "poverty of spirit," (Maté, 2022).

I wrote earlier about the loss of meaning in Amber's work life. I was experiencing an extreme existential dissatisfaction—an *existential crisis*. I didn't understand what I could possibly contribute to society in the future. Not only had I become disabled twenty years ago, I had also experienced a loss of identity when I could no longer work at my profession. I now had the loss of Amber to compound it. This feeling of uselessness was not just my obstacle. Society thought of women after menopause, Jackson said, as having outlived their ovaries, and outlived their usefulness as a human being. Jackson felt she might be just "marking time until [she] follows [her] glands into oblivion," (2021). I was feeling that I should have died, not Amber. I had less to offer. Without meaning, what was the point?

Meaning is so important in life, and when we lose meaning, we are at risk for disease. Kessler countered this thought with the belief that "if you occupy space on the planet, you have meaning," (2019). Kessler felt that hope has a very close relationship to meaning. *Hope* is what we need to find when grieving.

Around this time of prolonged grief, COVID-19 shut down the world, leaving us cowering in our homes, afraid we would get this terrible illness. It added to my loss of connection with others. We had already lost some contacts when Amber went to work and we were driving back and forth, and during the grieving, there was little connection at all. I had also become dislocated from myself. With "social dislocation," according to Bruce Perry, we become "cut off from autonomy, relatedness, trust, and meaning," (Maté, 2022). Any loss is trauma. Heath wrote that Post-Traumatic Stress Disorder can result in the feelings being re-triggered, making the person grieve again (2015). Some people suffer from unresolved grief in this manner. One in ten do not adjust over a long period and do not return to feeling they have meaningful lives. Prolonged grief is now in the Diagnostic and Statistical Manual for Mental Disorders (DSM5-TR). "Intense yearning, preoccupying thoughts of the deceased, intense emotional pain, feeling of disbelief, inability to accept loss, inability to engage or make plans, feeling that part of the self is lost," are all symptoms of prolonged grief. As each May came around, I would relive the days before Amber was admitted to the hospital. The time between May and mid-July was filled with these thoughts of her tortured existence at home without therapy. Helping Amber through the death process was traumatic for me. I had never experienced death up close. When my father died, I wasn't there because I was given the job of taking Mom for some lunch. My brother, David, had stayed at the hospital during the nights leading up to his death. Then, I would be re-triggered every holiday. Everything seemed so meaningless. Why bother with a celebration? My asthma made us remove the Christmas tree I lovingly decorated yearly. There was also Amber's birthday the day after mine. Pretty much all year long, it was filled with grief. It is one reason why I decided to write this book. If I wrote the story and we had something in our hands, not in my brain, maybe I could release it. Noting this story down was my way of hoping for healing. Writing this narrative has settled the grief somewhat. I think the narrative being in a concrete form allowed my brain to stop constantly ruminating. The brain was reassured that the memory of Amber would not be lost. James Pennebaker of the University of Texas found that people who would not tell about their trauma had higher rates of death, but if the story of trauma was written, it could improve their life. The best effect is possible when the story is handwritten. The story didn't need to be shared with anyone to gain the improvement (Kessler, 2019). The writing of the story affects us in three ways. The first is cause and effect. The second way is that the story can change our perspective. And the third way is by finding positive meaning of the experience. Amber's story has been told to myself and others frequently. Probably so frequently, it has burned its own pathway in my brain's neuro-structure.

Celebrations in our life after the death and COVID are much smaller. The loss of our beloved dog complicated the issue, and the memories of my father's unhappy death continued. My estrangement from my mother further complicated my feelings. I had experienced the loss of my mom years before her actual death and grieved this loss as well. The loss of Amber was the most important part of my grief. I am still not sure of my future. I have been really ill and fatigued of late, so I can't find a place where I can make a difference. I try to remember that I just have to "*be*," but like Amber, I seek meaning.

I also wrote the book to explore more about the risk factors that complicated Amber's life. I wanted to understand why this happened. I treated the story like a case study and examined all the questions that became evident for me. Amber had many risk factors, but it does not mean that is why she became ill. They are just all building blocks that may have complicated or advanced the carcinoma. No single item is the sole cause of a traumatic event. I discovered many risk factors that I had not been aware of. I am not blaming Amber for her illness. I think just living in today's world, the culture, the environment, the pollution, the job insecurity, and constant rejection when she looked for jobs all played a part, but may not be causative. Recently, I read that the distance from fuel refineries can affect cancer and I calculated if we were within that distance for most of the time that Amber was growing up. We were. I wasn't aware that living had an impact on dying. Maté described disease as often "being the result of millions of individual decisions at millions points of time." Disease is a process and also a "function of past generations of suffering, childhood trauma, of physiology, emotional histories, all acting within a physical and psychological environment," (2022). Disease may be genetic also. My exploration was sparked by what a friend of Amber's had said about how medicine treated women and the obese. I wondered why women were mistreated by medicine, and I wanted to know if Amber's friends were right about the bias against obesity in the medical field. I was shocked by what I learned. So, this book was also a learning experience for me. It became my own therapy, my own way of coping. I hope by sharing the risks, and Amber's story, that this might help others, furthering Amber's and my meanings in life.

EULOGY FROM A FRIEND
Written by Michelle Retterath

Amber loved an excellent horoscope and was always looking for signs from the universe, so when I went to yoga class a couple of days before she passed away, I couldn't help gasping when the teacher, who usually opened with a poem, instead started reading a recent post from astrologist Chani Nichols—one of Amber's heroes. It was about the upcoming eclipse season in the sign of Cancer, and Amber's last Chani post. Part of this says this: "We curate a well-lived life by developing and demonstrating our ability to care. If Eclipse Season teaches us anything, it's that it is in our best interest to direct our efforts toward what is most impactful. Ushering us into a time of personal growth, eclipses bridge the gap between our private and societal lives. What inhibits our access to the truth cuts away. Quickly."

Although I know Amber doubted herself, I hope that she saw these words as clear affirmation from the universe that she had lived her life well and fully accepted as truth that her life had meaning. That meaning grew out of her extraordinary capacity to care. Amber wanted to be a great artist and writer. She wanted to share ideas with fabulous people, make beautiful work, and write things that would open closed minds and improve the world. She did that, and her work will resonate far beyond the years that she got to live. But what

I hope she felt, too, was the other truth of her life, and that is the impact she had on the people who loved her. It's the many little things about Amber that I have been missing this week. Like her beautiful hair that I couldn't stop myself from complimenting even as she lay in her hospital bed and how she laughed. Or, the next I visited, the last time I ever saw her, how she took the time to tell me I looked nice that day, that she liked my dress. In a world where women so often cut each other down, I understood at that moment how much she and I had built each other up over the years. We wove so many little kindnesses into our conversation that they started to carry us all the time. We sought each other out when we needed a kinder take on ourselves. And Amber was one of the most intelligent people I ever knew, which was one of the reasons I trusted her opinion. Of course, she thought all her friends were as bright as her. I tried to tell her she was wrong (at least about me), but she would never hear it.

But she was also critical and unafraid to oppose ideas that distressed her. She was more interested in speaking her truth than being careful with other people's egos. It mattered more to her to fight for what she thought was correct than to ensure people liked her.

And just as she was willing to fight for the causes she believed in, she was ready to fight for her friends. A few years ago, a guy from my work met Amber at a party, and she said, "Kind of tore him a new one." After mentioning me, he responded, "Oh, does she walk with a limp?" I had to somewhat drag the story out of her because she didn't want me to feel bad, but I still find myself giggling about it whenever I think of her righteous anger aimed at an unsuspecting dude. I know that many of us already miss having Amber in our corner.

She believed that each of her friends was awesome and deserving of high-paying jobs, affordable and excellent housing, exciting dates, good sex, and endless love. And when the world disappointed me or my heart was broken, she would follow me into the dark and help me understand that there was nothing wrong with our romantic hearts. She fully understood and accepted the feelings and hopes that I was too embarrassed to share with others. She supported anything that would make her friends feel happy and free because even the idea that we might get what we wanted was enough to make her joyful, too. And I miss chatting with her every day. I want to tell her about all the days since August first. Most of all, I want to plan our next visit. Laughing with elbows on the table, hands around our beer pints or ten brunch coffee refills. She held my gaze and took the next sip so I would know she was still listening, but I had no doubt. She was generous with her attention and memory for every person, place, and thing I ever talked to her about. I rarely had to remind her who someone was or why they were important to me. And that's not just because her brain was a fantastic sponge. She cared. Just think about that for a second. How awesome it is to find someone who cares as much about your life as you do. However, it could also be because she loved a good story.

Amber loved romance novels and chick flicks with gushy endings. She had intense crushes and always dreamed of the future in elaborate detail. And if you ever had a beard, and you're good with your hands, and you can carry on an intelligent conversation about gender politics, she was probably in love with you at once or for all time. Bonus points if you go home and find that you're walking around with a little hole in your shirt all day. Looking at her, totally dreamy and adorable in your obliviousness and vulnerability.

Amber delighted in dreaming. And while some of her dreams sounded ordinary—like buying a great couch or having an apartment of her own, again—I know she would have reacted to these things as if they were extraordinary with all the gratitude and bliss that waited in her hopeful heart.

She absolutely believed that no person was no better than another. In particular, she knew and tried to help other people see that time is precious to everyone, and that a person's time and energy should be respected. When she wanted things for herself, it always seemed to turn into a broader statement or discussion on the state of the world. She didn't just want to be happy and live in lavish abundance HERSELF. She wanted that kind of joy and freedom for everyone.

When I got the news that Amber had passed away, I was surprised to find that I felt only peace at first. When I tuned into her energy, I understood why. It felt like she was happily surprised. Kind of like, "Oh, THIS is what death is? Okay!" And don't get me wrong, comforting as this was, I was still devastated. The first two weeks of August are a blur of shock and pain, and some of the most desperate crying I've ever done. But I also kept finding myself singing and listening to music outside my usual sad sack playlist. I danced a lot, especially in the morning, and I am not a morning person. And you can scoff. I really don't mind, but I danced because I felt that she was dancing. And laughing whenever I joined her.

When Amber was in pain, I just prayed for her to be at peace, but apparently the universe finally realized she deserved more because her energy since she passed on isn't just peaceful. It's blissful. I think she knows that we're the ones who need peace now. And I believe she is doing her best to bring it to everyone who loved her. I am so grateful that her kindness and generosity has extended even past her life and that she has helped me heal from the agony of this loss.

I hope that this resonates with some of you, if not because you've been dancing to the same songs, then because you have begun to find your own way to peace. Though I get the feeling Amber would like us all to aim for bliss. I think she would say that we deserve that because we are her friends, and her friends are awesome. Thank you.

BIBLIOGRAPHY

Didion, Joan, *The Year of Magical Thinking*, New York: Alfred A. Knopf, 2005, 2nd printing 2022.

Copaken, Deborah, *Ladyparts*, New York: Random House, 2021.

Dusenbury, Maya, *Doing Harm: The Truth About Bad Medicine and Lazy Science Leave Women Dismissed, Misdiagnosed, and Sick*, New York: HarperCollins, 2017.

Dresser, Sam, *How Not to Fear Your Death*, Aeon. (2020)

Dworkin, Andrea, *Intercourse,* New York: Basic Books 2007.

Findlay, Timothy, *Famous Last Words*, Toronto, Ont., Canada: Penguin, 2005.

Fung, Jason, *The Cancer Code: A Revolutionary New Understanding of a Medical Mystery*, New York: HarperCollins Publishers, 2020.

Atul Gawende, *Being Mortal*, March 2019

Hollis, James, *Finding Meaning in The Second Half of Life of Life: How to Finally, Grow Up*, Gotham Books, New York: Penguin Group, 2005.

Holt-Lunstad, J., Smith,T.B. and Layton,J. *Social Relationships and Mortality-Analytic Review,* PlosMedicine 7(7): e 1000316,doi.371/ journal.pmed 100031, 2010.

Jackson, Gabrielle, *Pain and Prejudice: How the Medical System Ignores Women and What To Do About It,* Vancouver, Canada: Greystone Books, 2019.

Jefferson, Margo. *A Construction of a Nervous System: A Memoir*, New York: Vintage Books, 2023.

Kalanithi, Paul, *When Breath Becomes Air*, Waterville, Maine: Thorndyke Press (large Print), 2016.

Kessler, David, *Finding Meaning: The Sixth Stage of Grief*. New York: Scribner, 2019.

Landgraff, Amber, *Relief Support*, Toronto, Ontario: Xpace Cultural Centre, OCADU, Vol.6., 2014-2015.

Landgraff, Amber, *It Happened in the Woods*, Toronto, Ontario: Xpace Cultural Centre, OCADU, Volume 3, 2011-2012.

Maté, Gabor with Maté, Daniel, *The Myth of Normal: Trauma, Illness and Healing in a Toxic Culture,* Toronto, Ontario: Alfred A. Knopf Canada, 2022.

Merton, Thomas, *The Seven Storey Mountain: An Autobiography,* Boston Maine: Mariner Books, 1999.

Moody, Raymond and Perry, Paul, *Proof of Life After Life*, New York: Atria Book, 2023.

Norman, Abby, *Ask Me About My Uterus: A Quest to make Doctors Believe in Women's Pain*, New York: Nation Books, 2018.

O'Connor, Frances, *The Grieving Brain: The Surprising Science of How We Learn from Love and Loss*, New York: HarperOne, 2022.

Puhl, Rebeca, *For Obese People, Prejudice is in Plain Sight*, The New York Times, March 5, 2010. www.nytimes.com/2010/03/16/healthy/16essa.html.

Umberson, Debra and Karas Montez, Jennifer. *A Flashpoint for Health Policy*, Journal of Health and Social Behavior, Aug 4,2011. ncbi.nih/prac/articles/PMC3150158.

Vafadis, Dorothea, *How Bias and Stigma Affects Patients,* 2022.

Van Tulleken, Chris, *Ultra Processed People: Why We Can't Stop Eating Food That Isn't Food,* Toronto, Ontario: Alfred E Knopf, 2023.

www.ingramcontent.com/pod-product-compliance
Lightning Source LLC
Chambersburg PA
CBHW070433290526
45791CB00005B/1963